DIGEST THIS

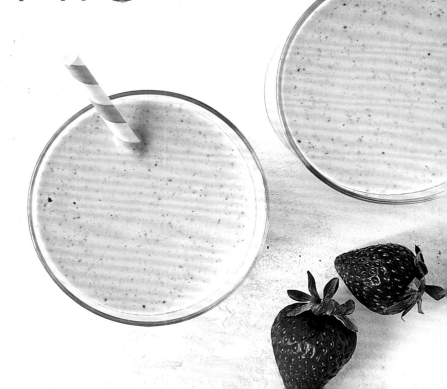

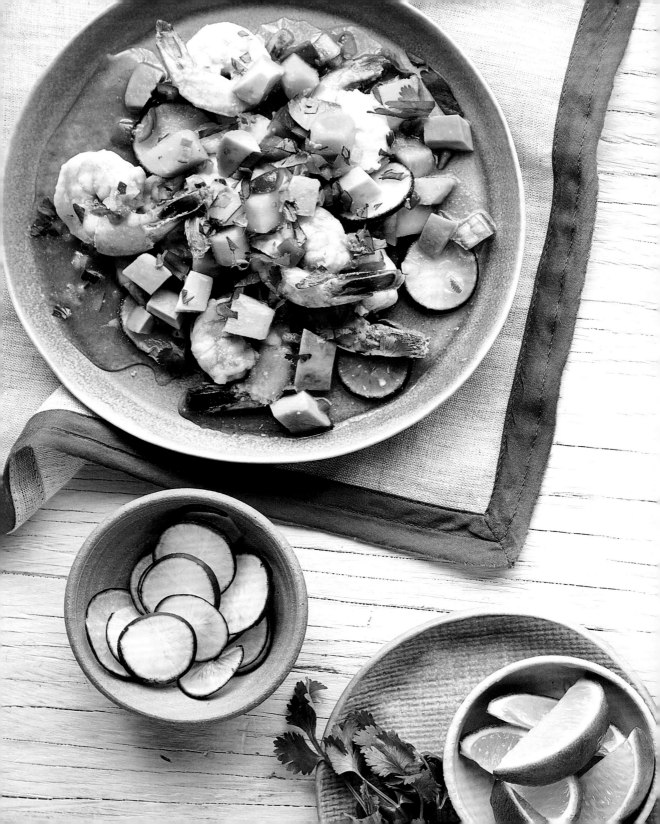

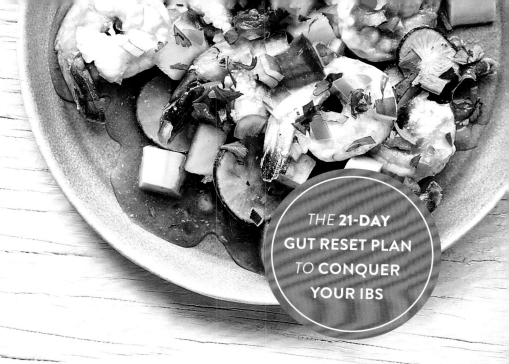

THE **21-DAY**
GUT RESET PLAN
TO **CONQUER**
YOUR IBS

DIGEST THIS

BETHANY UGARTE

RODALE.

Published in the United States by Rodale Books, an imprint of Random House, a division of Penguin Random House LLC, New York.
rodalebooks.com

RODALE and the Plant colophon are registered trademarks of Penguin Random House LLC.

Library of Congress Cataloging-in-Publication Data
Names: Ugarte, Bethany, author.
Title: Digest this : the 21-day gut reset plan to conquer your IBS / by Bethany Ugarte.
Description: New York : Rodale Books, 2020. | Includes index.
Identifiers: LCCN 2019057485 | ISBN 9780593136461 (trade paperback) | ISBN 9780593136478 (ebook)
Subjects: LCSH: Gastrointestinal system—Diseases—Diet therapy—Recipes. | Irritable colon—Diet therapy—Recipes. | Low-carbohydrate diet—Recipes. | Gastrointestinal system—Diseases—Alternative treatment—Popular works.
Classification: LCC RC819.D5 U33 2020 | DDC 641.5/6383—dc23
LC record available at https://lccn.loc.gov/2019057485

ISBN 978-0-593-13646-1
Ebook ISBN 978-0-593-13647-8

Printed in China

Book design by Jennifer K. Beal Davis
Cover and interior photographs by Hélène Dujardin
Cover design by Jennifer K. Beal Davis

10 9 8 7 6 5 4 3 2 1

First Edition

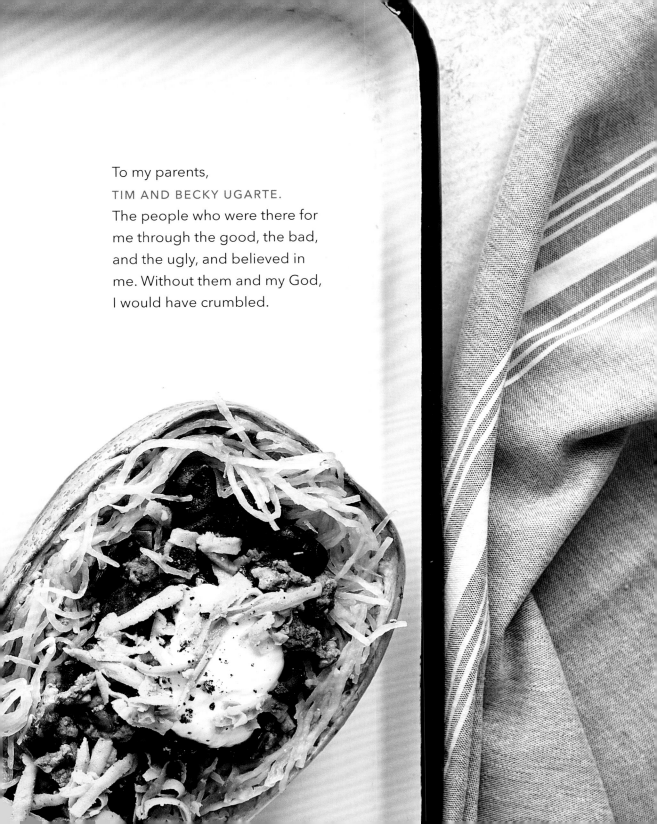

To my parents,
TIM AND BECKY UGARTE.
The people who were there for
me through the good, the bad,
and the ugly, and believed in
me. Without them and my God,
I would have crumbled.

CONTENTS

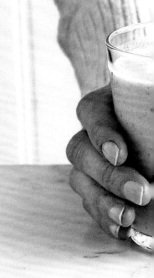

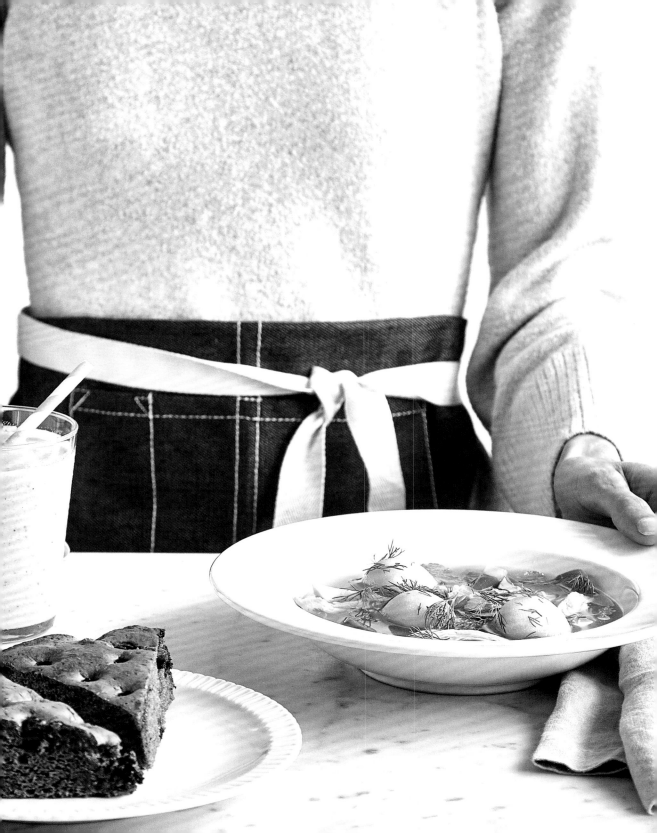

INTRODUCTION

No one really understands what it's like to have IBS, unless you have it yourself.

I know how it feels. And if you're reading this, you likely do, too. I suffered with its debilitating symptoms for years. I was bloated. I was gassy. I vomited frequently. I had constipation and diarrhea. I was constantly in the bathroom, and I had to miss work or regularly leave early. Eventually I even had to quit my dream job, because I was almost always in pain.

The irony? I've always loved food—and in fact I have been passionate about creating healthy, unique recipes that I've been sharing with hundreds of thousands of followers on Instagram for almost a decade. But all too often I couldn't eat the food I loved. Or if I did eat it, I got sick.

When you have IBS, or irritable bowel syndrome, you know what that feels like: the constant fear of what will happen if you eat something that triggers your symptoms. You worry every morning about whether you'll be okay today—whether you'll have to dash to the bathroom or cancel plans at the last minute because you're simply too sick to go.

You've been scared, frustrated, depressed, and angry. And if you're like a lot of (or let's face it, most) people, the "conventional" wisdom on how to treat IBS doesn't work for you. Doctors still don't understand exactly what causes IBS, so they typically suggest three basic strategies: change your diet, take drugs to manage your symptoms, and try not to be so stressed. Seriously. That's the typical "treatment."

I know this because, despite having just about every medical test you can imagine and seeing specialists throughout Los Angeles, including those in Beverly Hills and at top hospitals, I always heard the same thing. Avoid these foods. Or take these drugs. Or calm down. Or all three—but none of those strategies worked for me!

By the time I was in my early 20s, I was in so much pain that I could hardly eat . . . and what I did eat, I couldn't digest or absorb. My weight dropped from a healthy 125 pounds to 80 pounds. I was skeletal. I was bedridden. I couldn't leave the house.

But you know what? I got better. And so can you.

How did that happen? I bypassed the conventional wisdom. I knew quite a bit about digestive health already, and with the advice of a holistic doctor, I made some radical diet changes. I eliminated all gut irritants (and you may be amazed at how many things can irritate your gut—even "healthy" foods like beans, raw vegetables, and whole grains, not to mention common gums and fillers found in many processed foods), and I started consuming more protein, like grass-fed beef and organic chicken.

I pureed my protein (yes, that's right) to make it easier for my body to digest and absorb. I started eating plain, whole-milk cultured Greek yogurt to feed the probiotics, or healthy bacteria, in my gut. I created a drink that included specific digestive enzymes from different fruits and I drank it every day. I drank bone broth and took collagen and gelatin to help rebuild my gut. And most important, I stuck to the plan.

In less than a year—actually, in a matter of months—I healed my gut. Even better, I had developed a program that could (and has) worked for thousands of other people with IBS and other digestive issues—it was the basis of what would become this book. As one of the go-to experts on gut health on social media, I have hundreds of thousands of followers who rely on me for research-proven, crowd-tested advice.

Today, I'm free from the pain, bloating, and digestive issues I thought I was stuck with forever. I eat foods today my body couldn't handle before, because my gut is healthy and functioning the way it's supposed to. And I eat and enjoy my food without the fear of and worry about what may happen afterward.

My passion is developing recipes that are not only delicious and simple but also provide your gut with the nutrients it needs to heal. I can't say that I "cured" my IBS (I still have flare-ups now and then), but I can say that the program I developed did something that nothing else did. It restored my healthy gut function. And it just may do the same for yours.

No matter how miserable you feel, no matter how long you've been suffering, no matter how many different drugs or diets or plans you've tried for your IBS, I promise this plan will work for you. It may be unlike anything else you've heard of or seen before, but I and the thousands of readers who have road-tested these recipes can tell you, *it's what your gut needs.*

You may have spent years of your life suffering, but give yourself three weeks to try the Gut Reset, and you'll find that your life can and will change for the better. You'll no longer dread every morning and worry about how much pain or digestive problems you will have to deal with that day. You'll be free from discomfort, from fear, from the frustration you may have grown accustomed to . . . and you'll be free to look forward to and embrace not only food again but also your whole life.

If you're not that sick, you may not need to embark on the 21-day Gut Reset. But you'll still benefit from the recipes I've included here, which are simple to make and are loaded with nutrients that help your gut, as well as the rest of your body, function at its best. Whether your gut needs a complete overhaul or simply some fine-tuning, or even if you're just looking for the worry-free, flavor-bomb recipes, I'm here to help. So let's get started!

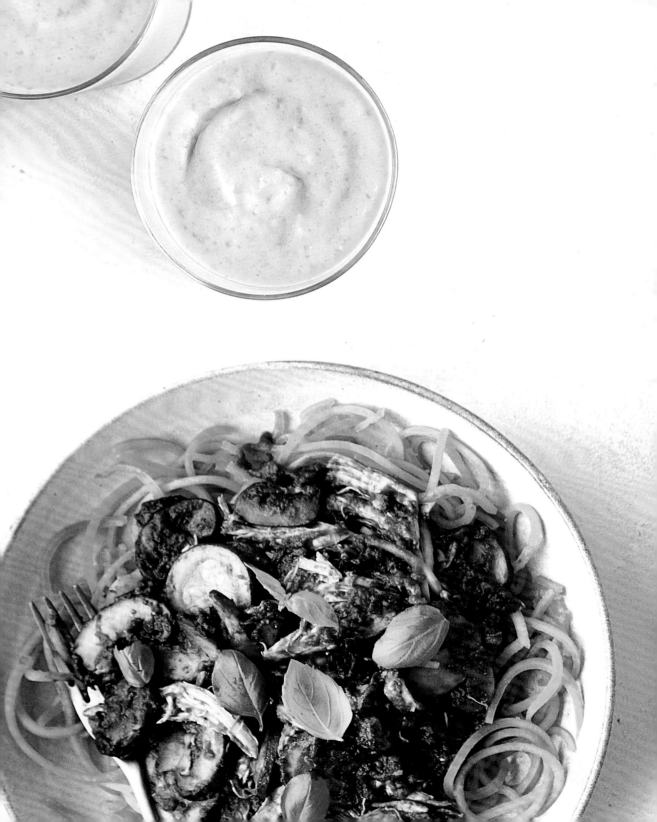

THE
DIGEST
THIS
PLAN

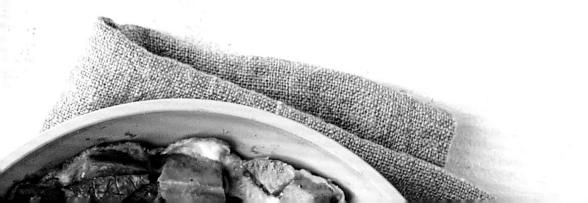

IT'S NOT IN YOUR HEAD— IT'S YOUR GUT

You may be trying to hide your IBS or digestive issues from coworkers, friends, or even your family, but you should know that you're not alone. As many as one in five Americans has irritable bowel syndrome (IBS), and that number appears to be on the rise. Plus, millions more struggle with gut problems on a regular basis (that keep them irregular!).

I'm here to tell you that IBS is not "all in your head." It doesn't mean you have occasional bouts of stomach upset or diarrhea. Rather, IBS is a chronic, debilitating disease that affects the lower GI tract and causes symptoms like abdominal pain, bloating, constipation, and diarrhea; it's also the most common gastrointestinal condition throughout the world.

It's one thing to say that the symptoms include diarrhea, constipation, bloating, and pain—blah, blah, blah. It's another thing to experience those symptoms on a daily basis, for years, even for decades. I know, because I did! IBS made me so sick that at one point I couldn't even leave my house. I had to quit my job; I'd lost 40 pounds, and I sometimes prayed to die because I didn't want to live through the daily pain. I was *that* sick and *that* miserable. And plenty of people are just as sick with IBS.

IBS, in a word, sucks. And it's not just me who thinks so!

Check this out:

- **IBS is painful.** When questioned, more than half of people with it—53 percent—have moderate pain and another 31 percent say it's severe. More than half of people with IBS have moderate bloating; 28 percent say their bloating is severe. Three-quarters of people experience moderate or severe diarrhea, and more than half (57 percent) have moderate or severe constipation.

- **IBS is difficult, sometimes impossible, to control.** Most people feel unable to manage their IBS symptoms—just one in five say their symptoms are under control. More than 70 percent find that their IBS symptoms interfere with everyday life; 46 percent have missed school or work due to IBS.

- **IBS is often misdiagnosed.** Many people with IBS try to manage the condition on their own, without seeking medical treatment. But when they do, they're often misdiagnosed. Up to four in ten may be diagnosed, not with IBS but instead with something like depression, stress/anxiety, food allergies, lactose intolerance, or GERD (gastroesophageal reflux, or acid reflux). (Complicating matters is the fact that depression and anxiety are both linked to IBS and may make you more likely to develop the condition. The reverse is true, too—simply having IBS makes you more likely to have depression and anxiety. It's a lose-lose situation!).

- **IBS is frustrating.** I know this because I've been blogging about my struggle with IBS and gut health for years, and I've heard from thousands of people who have described how hopeless and lost they feel. And surveys reveal that after their initial diagnosis, six in ten people worry that they'll never find a way to manage their symptoms, while 38 percent are frightened of the negative impact it will have on their social and family lives. And it does have an impact—a big one. Forty-six percent of people with IBS say that their symptoms "sometimes" interfere with work, school, and social situations; another 30 percent claim that their symptoms often or always interfere with their day-to-day life. Nearly 80 percent of people with IBS say they can't control their symptoms, and almost 40 percent worry constantly about when their symptoms will return. It's a miserable way to live.

- **IBS is isolating.** Many people suffer for years—and never even see a doctor for their symptoms. Up to 40 percent of people with these kinds of symptoms—that's literally millions—don't seek medical care and instead try to treat it on their own. (Of course, that's one reason I have so many followers on Instagram—people are looking for resources to heal themselves, and they are often desperate to find something that will work for them.)

HOW DO YOU KNOW IT'S IBS?

Can you relate to Brianne's story on the next page? Do you feel alone or misunderstood because of your digestive issues? Even though IBS is common, doctors still don't seem to "get" it. I think that's why so many people are misdiagnosed. Looking back, I know now that I suffered from IBS and some other digestive health conditions, like yeast overgrowth and gastroparesis, for more than a decade—yet doctors couldn't tell me what was wrong with me!

By the time I was in my mid-20s, I had abdominal pain, bloating, diarrhea, vomiting, gas, brain fog, and fatigue that were so severe and so uncontrollable that I had to quit my dream job. I was in constant pain, unable to work, and was barely able to get out of bed. My body lost the ability to digest food

BRIANNE'S STORY: STRESSING OVER FAMILY EVENTS AND GATHERINGS

I remember having GI issues as young as 12. I would get upset stomachs very easily, and at this time GI issues weren't really a common issue for young people so it was always just brushed off as "no big deal." As I got older it got worse, and my doctor couldn't find anything physically wrong so he prescribed some kind of antacid.

Later in my life, as a young adult, my issues just progressively got worse and I began to seek more medical attention. I've had upper GIs, a couple of upper endoscopies, blood work, and allergy testing. At 25, I was misdiagnosed with an autoimmune disease called "eosinophilic gastritis." My new GI doctor finally diagnosed me with IBS with specific food triggers two years later.

When I was young, my symptoms started with bloating and cramping with diarrhea or loose stool. Then it progressed to nausea with cramping and pains. Eventually the nausea got so severe that it prevented me from going to school at times. I remember calling myself in sick sometimes during junior high because I couldn't get out of the fetal position in my bed. Or I would lie there with a garbage can next to my bed for hours, feeling so sick. I worked in a salon for a few years in my early adulthood and would miss work frequently due to the severity of my symptoms (nausea, severe bloating, diarrhea, cramping, sharp pains). They only got worse as I got older. Sometimes flare-ups would last days at a time. During these flare-ups I wouldn't eat very much because I was so sick and would lose weight.

One year it got pretty bad, and my doctor was concerned about how much weight I had lost and how consistently it was coming off due to the struggle with my symptoms. During this time, I was so desperately just trying to determine what foods were causing these symptoms so that I could avoid them. It took me about a year before I figured it out.

I have struggled with anxiety and depression due to my struggle with my GI issues. I stress over normal events like family gatherings and birthday dinners, and parties or vacations, because I am so limited with my diet to "good foods." Most of our life events revolve around food and meals, and I have to put so much more thought and planning into what I'm going to eat. It is also extremely difficult explaining my situation to other people who have no GI issues.

I always get strange looks when I have to remove half the ingredients from an entree at a restaurant. I hate the feeling that I'm being judged about something I can't control. It just feels like people assume it's a choice, or that I have a weird relationship with food. My stepmom even tried to convince my dad that I had an eating disorder and that I was doing this to myself.

—Brianne, 28

and absorb nutrients, and my weight plummeted from a healthy 125 pounds to just 80. I literally looked like I was dying. And I was.

You name the medical procedure, I had it. Endoscopy. Colonoscopy. I had MRIs, blood work, stool samples, and urine samples. Breath tests and X-rays. CT scans, ultrasounds, food-sensitivity tests, and gastric-emptying tests. At one point, I was at the emergency room once a month because I was in such pain—yet nothing helped ease my symptoms. By 2016, all that doctors could tell me was that I "had IBS." I was offered prescriptions, was told to do yoga, urged to go gluten-free, get off dairy. I received no real answers.

IBS is a diagnosis "of exclusion," which means there's no definitive medical test for it. Your doctor may diagnose you with it after ruling out other potential conditions. Or you may have done your own research and determined that it must be IBS causing your digestive symptoms.

Doctors classify IBS into three categories:

- **IBS with constipation (IBS-C).** This is when your irregular bowel habits include constipation at least a quarter of the time. A diet that lacks fiber is thought to be a contributing cause.

- **IBS with diarrhea (IBS-D).** This is when your irregular bowel habits include diarrhea at least a quarter of the time. Diet is again considered a causative factor.

- **IBS with mixed bowel habits (IBS-M).** This is when your irregular bowel habits include constipation at least a quarter of the time and diarrhea at least a quarter of the time.

However, I can tell you that the type of IBS you have doesn't really matter. It doesn't even matter whether you've actually had a diagnosis of IBS! If your gut is out of whack, as I like to say, you're going to be miserable.

GETTING DIAGNOSED WITH IBS

So, let's say you've been dealing with gut issues for months now, maybe even years. You've got diarrhea, bloating, pain, constipation, fatigue. Your symptoms are severe enough to interfere with your life, so you do what most people do—you go to a doctor.

What happens next? Your doctor talks to you about your symptoms and performs an exam. She'll check for abdominal bloating and may feel your abdomen to see if you have tenderness or pain in the area. She'll ask you about your medical history and may order certain tests to help her rule out other conditions.

Your doc will want to know if you have a family history of digestive diseases. She'll also ask about your diet and whether you've noticed if certain foods seem to make your symptoms worse. She'll want to know what kinds of medications (both prescription and over-the-counter) you take, whether you've been sick recently, and whether you've dealt with any major stressful events recently. (Stress is a known trigger for IBS and it also makes the condition worse if you have already have it.)

Your doctor may take a blood sample or stool sample (or both) to check for conditions like anemia and inflammatory bowel disease. She may order other tests like a hydrogen breath test, which can determine whether you're lactose-intolerant. If your symptoms include heartburn, nausea, and vomiting or pain, she may order a test called an upper gastrointestinal ("GI") endoscopy, where a specialist uses an endoscope, which is a tiny camera on the end of a flexible tube, to look at the lining of the top part of your GI tract. This test can diagnose gastroesophageal reflux disease (GERD), celiac disease, Barrett's esophagus, cancer, and other conditions. She may also order a colonoscopy to look at the inside of your rectum and colon; this test can diagnose ulcers, polyps, and cancer.

But even if you have all these tests, your doctor can't say with absolute certainty if it is IBS. Ruling out other conditions, however, does make it more likely that IBS is the cause.

Remember, there's no simple test to determine whether you have IBS. Doctors look for symptoms that include:

- Abdominal pain that is related to bowel movements. That may mean that going to the bathroom either makes your pain worse or eases the pain.

- You're having bowel movements more frequently, or less frequently, than you used to.

- Your stools look different from how they did before. You may notice that you have loads of "gel" in your stool. This is mucus and/or intestinal lining. We all produce mucus to some degree and we all "shed" intestinal lining, but normally that's a gradual process, just like we shed outer skin constantly and regain new skin. However, when you can actually see the mucus or gel, this is the result of an autoimmune response and your body is attacking itself. You may even see un-digested food—yes, whole food—in your stool, and that's clearly not a good sign. It means your body is not digesting food, and ultimately not absorbing nutrients.

- You've had symptoms at least once a week during the last three months, or your symptoms started more than six months ago.

If you have several of these symptoms, and your doctor rules out other possible causes, he or she may tell you that you have IBS. Even if you don't have a formal diagnosis, though, these kinds of symptoms are a clear sign that your digestive system needs help. After all, you don't need a doctor to tell you if you're in pain or in the bathroom constantly, or that you feel miserable. You already know that.

GETTING A DIAGNOSIS OF IBS COSTS PLENTY

Simply attempting to get a diagnosis for IBS or other digestive issues can be expensive, according to a 2016 study from the medical journal *Clinical Therapeutics*.

Researchers found that doctors may prescribe tests including lab tests like thyroid and liver function; C-reactive protein, or CRP; erythrocyte sedimentation rate, or ESR; celiac panel; and complete blood count, or CBC. Procedures included endoscopy, hydrogen breath test, and abdominal or pelvic tomography (CT) scans. Researchers found that blood tests were performed in 49 percent of people diagnosed with IBS, while nearly half (47 percent) had imaging and endoscopic procedures performed. Nearly one in five, or 18 percent, had a sigmoidoscopy. Researchers found that IBS was the reason for 3.5 million doctor visits, even though a minority (between 10 and 25 percent) of people with IBS sought medical treatment for their symptoms. Another study found that the direct and indirect costs of IBS was *$20 billion* a year.

AMENA'S STORY: YOU DON'T HAVE TO BE DIAGNOSED WITH IBS TO BE MISERABLE

I was never officially diagnosed with IBS, but ever since my late teens I would have intense cramps and digestive issues after eating most foods. I was much more sensitive to all food (no allergies, though) compared to my three siblings. I was overweight, so I always ate diet foods and low-cal or low-fat foods.

My stomach issues and cramps definitely made me miss out on various work, school, and social events. It was embarrassing and painful, so I didn't want to be around people until a flare-up calmed down again. This affected me emotionally because I'm an extrovert and love people.

At first, to treat it, I cut out processed/packaged food and anything that obviously had any type of artificial sweetener (diet products, low-carb treats). That helped a little with cramps but was not enough. I still had intense pain and bowel irregularities.

—**Amena, 30**

IS THERE A BLOOD TEST FOR IBS?

There is still no definitive test for IBS. But here's something cool: a new company has developed a blood test that claims to help determine whether you have it. Researchers found that people with two types of IBS (IBS-D and IBS-M) have elevated levels of two antibodies—anti-CdtB and anti-vinculin—in their blood. (I'm not going to get all science-y on you, but basically the reverse seems to be true as well—if you have elevated levels of these antibodies, you've got one of those types of IBS.)

According to the company that developed it, the ibs-smart™ test determines how much of these two antibodies are in your blood, and estimates the likelihood of having IBS-D or IBS-M. It may be too early to ascertain how accurate this test is, but it's a sign that doctors are looking for a definitive test (finally!) for this condition. Talk to your doctor if you want to know more about this test; or check out https://www.ibssmart.com for more information about it.

Even if you have health insurance, it may not cover all the costs for these common tests—and if you don't have health insurance, you probably can't even afford most of these tests. According to the study, some of the most common tests involved in an IBS diagnosis include:

TEST AVERAGE COST

IBS diagnostic blood panel: $500

CBC (complete blood count): $149

Colonoscopy: $2,727

Upper endoscopy: $1,375

Computed tomography scan: $2,175

Ultrasound: $371

YOU'VE GOT IBS? NOW WHAT?

Getting diagnosed with IBS might seem like the hard part, but the crazy thing is that there's little advice out there on how to treat it (forget curing it!). Currently there are three approaches to treating IBS: dietary changes, such as avoiding FODMAPs (see next page) or other foods that make IBS worse; implementing stress-management techniques; or prescribing a variety of drugs (ranging from antibiotics to laxatives to antispasmodics to antidepressants) to help ease symptoms. Let's look at each approach:

CHANGE YOUR DIET

Dietary modifications are often the first line of attack when it comes to treating IBS. If constipation is one of your symptoms, consuming more fiber may help make it easier to go to the bathroom. However, adding too much fiber to your diet too quickly can backfire and make symptoms even worse. Avoiding gluten, a type of protein found in foods containing wheat, rye, and barley, may also help.

But the most common dietary recommendation is to follow a low FODMAP diet. FODMAP (which stands for fermentable oligosaccharides, disaccharides, monosaccharides, and polyols) are types of carbohydrates that can be difficult to digest. FODMAP foods include:

- Milk and other dairy products, including soft cheeses, yogurt, and ice cream

- Wheat products

- Fruits like apples, apricots, blackberries, cherries, mangoes, nectarines, pears, plums, and watermelons

- Vegetables, including artichokes, asparagus, beans, cabbage, cauliflower, garlic and garlic salts, lentils, mushrooms, onions, and sugar snap or snow peas

- Canned fruit, dried fruit, and fruit juices

- Honey and foods containing high-fructose corn syrup

- Artificial sweeteners like sorbitol, mannitol, xylitol, and maltitol

Following a low FODMAP diet that eliminates these foods has been shown to help some people's IBS symptoms. And that's great if it works for you. However, all this diet does is help you avoid gut irritants, and it doesn't help everyone with IBS. In addition, there may be other non-FODMAP foods that bother your gut but may not bother someone else's, and vice versa.

I tried eliminating most FODMAP foods myself and went vegan, but that didn't help me. Actually, when I tried a vegan diet, it seemed to make things worse, but I was desperate to try anything at that point. As I found out, though, to finally get better I had to heal my gut with the right foods instead of just eliminating these gut irritants.

TAKE MEDICINES THAT HELP

We're a country that seems to believe that the solution to any kind of medical problem is to take a pill, so it's not surprising that many doctors push medications to treat IBS. These medications range from antidiarrhea medicine to laxatives to antidepressants. Yet these medicines don't always work, and some people (me included!) don't want to have to rely on drugs to feel better. And that's not just because of the cost of these meds or the side effects they may cause.

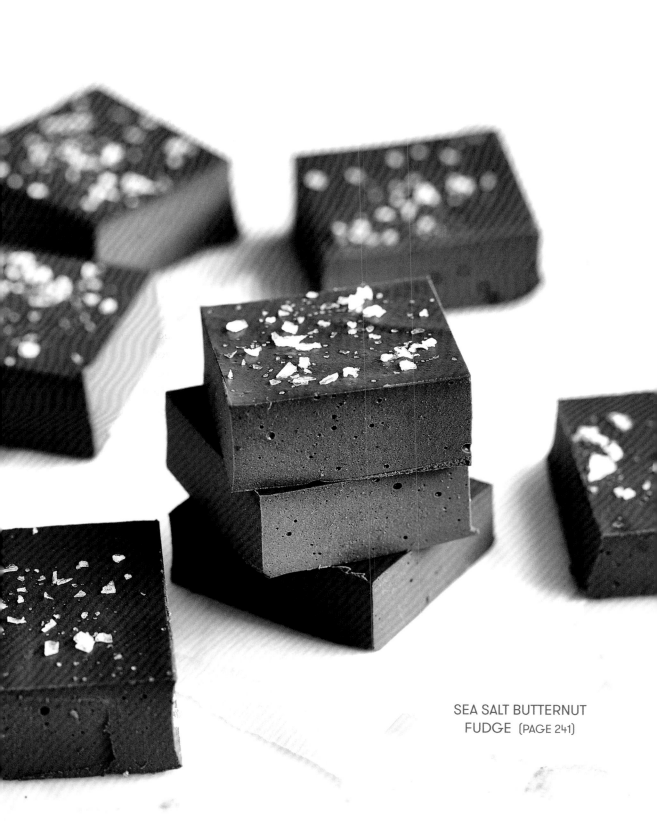

SEA SALT BUTTERNUT
FUDGE (PAGE 241)

COMMON MEDICATIONS USED TO TREAT IBS

Not feeling well? There's a pill that will make you feel better—or so the pharmaceutical industry would have you believe. Nearly half of all adults have taken at least one prescription medication in the last 30 days alone.

Many doctors' first line of treatment for IBS symptoms is to prescribe medication along with dietary changes. These medications may ease symptoms, but none of them helped me—nor do I recommend them to others. (But I'm not a doctor, so please keep that mind!) According to the National Institute of Diabetes and Digestive and Kidney Diseases, some of the most common medicines used to treat IBS symptoms include:

- **Alosetron.** This medication treats diarrhea, cramping, and urgency, and is prescribed only to women.
- **Antidepressants.** Low doses of drugs like selective serotonin reuptake inhibitors are often prescribed and may help ease IBS symptoms, likely because of the gut/brain connection you'll learn about next.

- **Antispasmodics.** These drugs reduce muscle spasms and can help alleviate cramping and diarrhea.
- **Eluxadoline.** This prescription medication decreases bowel activity.
- **Linaclotide.** This drug helps speed the movement of food and waste through the digestive system.
- **Loperamide.** This antidiarrhea medicine is available in both over-the-counter and prescription versions.
- **Lubiprostone.** This prescription laxative helps produce softer, more frequent bowel movements and can reduce stomach pain and bloating. It's used to treat irritable bowel syndrome with constipation, and is usually prescribed to women.
- **Plecanatide.** Like linaclotide, this medicine helps increase the movement of food and waste through the digestive system.
- **Rifaximin.** This antibiotic kills bacteria in the intestine that can cause diarrhea.

MANAGE STRESS BETTER

Because of the clear connection between stress and IBS, lifestyle changes are often suggested as a treatment for IBS. That includes doing things like getting more sleep (and better-quality sleep), exercising more frequently, and avoiding stress when you can. Your doctor may suggest cognitive behavioral therapy, gut-directed hypnotherapy (a form of hypnosis to treat intestinal symptoms), or relaxation training.

Again, however, the advice that doctors often give can be vague or prove difficult to follow. Maybe you don't have the time or the money to pursue therapy. And it's pretty much impossible to avoid all stress, especially when you're dealing with painful, unpredictable IBS symptoms! So the question becomes: *How can you effectively manage your stress?* (Don't worry—we're going to talk *lots* more about this later in the book. I'll show you ways to de-stress, which in turn will help your symptoms.)

YOUR SECOND BRAIN AND HOW IT WORKS

I don't want to say that sometimes doctors are wrong . . . but, hey, sometimes they are. I didn't get better until I rejected a lot of conventional advice about how to treat IBS and created the radical *Digest This* plan (including the 21-day Gut Reset) that you'll learn more about in a bit. But before we get into that, let's talk about the relationship between your gut and your brain.

Your digestive tract is called the "second brain" for a reason. Your gut, which includes the small and large intestines, includes bacteria (also called "gut flora" or microbiome) that help break down the nutrients in the food you eat into smaller particles that your body can use for energy.

When your gut is healthy, that process is seamless. When you have a condition like IBS, however, your body can't digest and metabolize food properly, and the result is a multifaceted list of symptoms, including:

- gas
- pain
- bloating
- diarrhea
- constipation
- nutrient malabsorption/malnutrition
- brain fog
- fatigue
- depression
- bowel obstruction
- interference with normal hunger/fullness signals
- feeling like you have to "go" even after you've gone to the bathroom

Just as there is no definitive test for IBS, researchers still don't know the exact cause of IBS. However, they suspect it may be due to a problem with the brain–gut interaction (how your brain and gut work together). Your brain and your gut communicate with each other—they "talk" to each other all the time. That means if your gut is malfunctioning, it may affect your brain health as well, impacting the neurotransmitters that affect mood.

This may explain the link between IBS and anxiety and depression, and why people with IBS are more likely to have either or both conditions. From a positive standpoint, this means that healing your gut may also have an impact on your mental health and could help ease depression and anxiety.

We could not know the cause, but we know that certain factors may increase your risk of developing IBS, including:

- a stressful or unhappy childhood
- a traumatic event suffered at a young age
- some mental disorders, including depression and anxiety
- bacterial infections of the digestive tract
- overgrowth of bacteria in the small intestine (more about gut bacteria in the next couple of chapters)
- food intolerances or sensitivities
- a history of dieting
- over-exercising/failing to take enough rest days
- a genetic propensity to develop the condition

Note that some of these factors, like a stressful childhood or an anxiety disorder, are related to your mental health, while others involve the health and functioning of your gut. And you probably already have experienced firsthand that feeling stressed out or upset makes your symptoms worse. Whenever I get stressed out, have too much on my plate, feel like there's just too much going on in the day, or if something didn't go as planned, my digestion certainly acts up. And not just for a few minutes. For hours, even days, my gut is a wreck . . . all because I allowed my emotions and mental state to get the better of me.

Other times, a hard workout can cause a flare. I used to work out every day, for hours. I was addicted! Sure, it made me feel good the first hour and gave me that endorphin rush we all crave, but I didn't realize that I was overdoing it—or how much all that exercise was affecting my nervous system and my brain.

DEALING WITH IBS ON A DAY-TO-DAY BASIS

That's enough about what *causes* IBS! There's not much you can do about your childhood, or whether you have food intolerances or have had food poisoning, after all. Let's switch gears and talk about the things that can make IBS symptoms worse. (And if you feel like the answer to that is "everything," I get it! I've felt the same way.)

CONSUMING DAIRY PRODUCTS, FOODS CONTAINING GLUTEN, OR HIGH-FAT FOODS

Here's the thing: If your body can't properly break down food, you're going to have symptoms like gas, bloating, and diarrhea. You may know if you have a dairy allergy, but you can be sensitive to gluten and never identify it as a problem because you're eating it all the time. Even if you don't have food intolerances, foods high in fat are hard to digest. (Side note: Avocados are good for you because of the healthy, monounsaturated fat they contain, but I personally had a hard time digesting avocados for a long time. I had to work up a tolerance to them, but thankfully I can now eat avocados and other healthy fats and you'll be able to, too! So have hope!)

CARBONATED BEVERAGES, CAFFEINE, AND ALCOHOL

Carbonated bevvies can make you gassy and uncomfortable, and caffeine and alcohol can dehydrate you, making you feel nauseous, constipated, and headachy.

CAN FOOD POISONING CAUSE IBS?

Ever had food poisoning? It's a relatively common condition, affecting about 15 percent of people every year. Well, did you know that even one instance of food poisoning may increase your risk of developing IBS? A review that looked at more than 40 studies found that more than 45 percent of people with food poisoning later developed IBS.

This conclusion showed that there was a four times higher risk of developing IBS compared to people who hadn't had food poisoning. Women were more likely to develop IBS after food poisoning than men, and people who had used antibiotics were also more likely to develop it. Even one bout of food poisoning appears to alter the microbiome in the gut enough to set up a person for IBS.

That's scary, but fortunately you can improve your gut health, even if you've had food poisoning—or you get it in the future.

STRESS

I know, I know—who isn't stressed? But if you have IBS or gut issues, you're likely to experience symptoms as a result. Remember the gut-brain connection? The more stressed you are, the worse your symptoms are likely to be—unless you find healthy ways of managing that stress. I use different ways to de-stress depending on the day. Sometimes a good workout helps; other days, not working out and just taking a nap calms me down. More often than not, cleaning my house helps! Huh? If you're like me, having a dirty house, seeing piles of laundry, and having loads of dishes to wash actually make me stressed! So, keeping a clean house helps me "breathe" a little. I also take CBD (cannabidiol), which has also been a huge factor in taking the edge off of stress. It mainly helps me sleep—and when you get a good night's sleep, that's when your body, your gut, and your brain can recharge and heal.

HORMONAL CHANGES (SUCH AS DURING YOUR MENSTRUAL CYCLE)

Do your IBS symptoms tend to follow your cycle? I know mine do. First off, lots of women have GI symptoms—bloating, abdominal pain, diarrhea, constipation—that correlate to where they are in their cycle. Pain and diarrhea tend to be more common in the first half of your cycle (before ovulation), while bloating and constipation are worse in the second half of your cycle, and those hormonal changes often aggravate your IBS symptoms. If you have IBS, you're also more likely to have painful periods, cramping, and premenstrual syndrome than women without it.

DRUGS, INCLUDING ANTIBIOTICS

Antibiotics kill bacteria, which means that these medications can affect the microbiome, throwing it out of whack (more about antibiotics in the next chapter).

EATING TOO QUICKLY OR WHILE DISTRACTED

How often do you eat while you're checking Instagram, watching TV, or sitting at your desk? Constantly, right? Well, our bodies are not meant to digest food when we're preoccupied, rushed, or stressed; that distraction interferes with normal digestion, even in people without IBS. But if you have IBS, rushing through a meal is likely to make you feel sick just minutes later. (I admit with a busy schedule like mine, I tend to eat while working to "save time," but whenever I sit down with no technology and no work, I feel much better after my meal.)

Eating while talking is also another factor. For instance, when you're out to eat with a friend and you feel "rushed" during the meal because you're trying to hold a conversation, and the only way to do that is to eat super fast (mostly likely not chewing all the way and swallowing large pieces of food) so you can then talk. Or there's chewing while talking—this actually creates gas!

A LACK OF EXERCISE

You already know that exercise is good for you, but it also helps your digestive tract function properly. If you're sedentary, your digestion may be sluggish as well. But here's the problem—when your IBS symptoms are out of control, you may be in too much pain to even go for a walk. And who wants to go to the gym when you don't know if you'll need to rush to the bathroom? And that does not even mention the fact that exercising, or exercising too much, can also make IBS worse. It depends on you as a person and your history of exercise.

POOR SLEEP HABITS

Just like exercise, a lack of sleep or a lack of quality sleep can make IBS symptoms worse. But once again, if you're up half the night in the bathroom, your sleep is going to suffer!

ANXIETY AND FEAR RELATED TO WHAT YOU'RE EATING

In other words, yes—just worrying about IBS can make your IBS worse! This is a HUGE one for me! I used to worry when the holidays came around. On Thanksgiving Day, I would be so nervous about eating in front of others because I felt pressured to do so. I didn't want to be the odd one out, and I didn't want to offend anyone if I failed to sample their dish or have people think I wasn't eating. Fact was, I couldn't eat the food everyone else was eating! But people just didn't understand. All this gave me huge anxiety. I ended up not eating anything, and still I had an upset stomach for some reason (probably from the anxiety). After years of this pattern, I finally gave up caring what others thought and I brought my own food to eat. After a while, my family got used to it, and they learned to understand why I had to do what I did. And years later, I came to find out that they really didn't even care if I ate differently! Thankfully I can now venture out into sampling more foods as my gut has healed significantly, but back then I had to make my own food—and not give a hoot!

DON'T GIVE UP—THE GOOD NEWS (AND IT'S *REALLY* GOOD NEWS!)

That's the bad news—and there's a lot of it. But what's the good news? No matter how severe your symptoms may be, you *can* begin the process of healing your gut in just 21 days with my Gut Reset program. This program works for people with IBS and other gut issues, even when nothing else does—including diet changes, medications, and stress management. The program is simple in structure; it's based on avoiding all gut irritants and consuming the foods that your gut needs to "heal and seal" itself.

Here's a quick preview of what to expect. First, you'll eliminate all gut irritants from your diet, and you'll rely instead on foods that help heal your gut. You do this for 21 days. I call this the Gut Reset, and unlike traditional diet plans tailored for IBS, it will calm even the most irritated gut while providing your body with the nutrients it desperately needs. During this time you'll eat foods like full-fat cultured yogurt, pureed protein, and all kinds of delicious smoothies. And in just 21 days, your gut will be the healthiest it's been in months, possibly in years. That's because these simple but nutrient-dense foods are easy for your gut to digest. They help reduce inflammation and introduce ingredients like collagen and gelatin to help repair the holes in your gut, as well as help reset your gut to a healthy balance.

After the 21-day Gut Reset, you are free to include other foods to maintain the plan for healing. I do encourage you to experiment and see if your gut can handle foods that may have been major triggers before. But how you'll react to these foods will depend on how long you've had IBS symptoms, how damaged your gut is, and how far along you are in the healing process. In short, the longer you've had IBS, the longer it may take your gut to completely heal.

And that's it! There are no phases or programs or restrictions after you finish the 21-day Gut Reset, although you'll want to avoid foods that you know make your symptoms worse. But you may find after healing your gut that you're now able to eat foods that may have triggered symptoms before. You won't know until you try!

And if you're reading this and thinking, *Okay, well, my symptoms aren't that bad . . . but I still want to feel better overall,* you can skip the 21-day Gut Reset and just enjoy the recipes you'll find in this book. (I hope you'll at least consider trying the Gut Reset, though, because your gut can do a *lot* of healing when you provide it with these calming foods in this relatively short period.)

Specifically, my program is based on the following eight principles:

- **Principle #1:** Eat pureed protein every day. You puree the protein to predigest it, which makes it easier for your body to break down and absorb.

- **Principle #2:** Eat plain, whole-milk cultured Greek yogurt (preferably with rice, which helps the probiotics in the yogurt survive to the digestive tract). The probiotics in yogurt will help build up the healthy bacteria in your gut.

- **Principle #3:** Every morning, consume a Digestive Boost (page 101), a fruit enzyme drink consisting of papaya, pineapple, mango, and kiwi.

- **Principle #4:** Consume bone broth every day. It's loaded with gut-building nutrients.

- **Principle #5:** Consume only foods that are included in the Gut Reset program—that includes all the smoothie recipes in chapter 7. They are free from all gut irritants and contain the nutrients that your gut needs to heal.

- **Principle #6:** Consume gelatin, collagen, and/or L-glutamine every day, which helps create healthy gut walls and promotes a healthier gut overall.

- **Principle #7:** Turn on the parasympathetic nervous system before you eat. This means no more eating while driving, checking social media, working, or doing anything else—except slowing down and focusing on your food.

- **Principle #8:** Perform at least one stress-reduction technique every day. Learn how to enhance the brain-gut connection by managing your stress, no matter how demanding or challenging your life is.

That's it—the entirety of the Gut Reset program. And yes, you will have to give up your regular way of eating for 21 days and do some things that may seem weird (like pureeing your chicken), but if you're willing to stick with it, it will work. You'll be free of the symptoms that have plagued you, and you will learn how to eat for the rest of your life so as to maintain your newly healed gut.

Better still, you'll find dozens of easy-to-prepare, tasty recipes that are good for your gut and the rest of your body. And even if your symptoms aren't serious enough to require a critical intervention like the 21-day Gut Reset, have no worries: By following my general *Digest This* maintenance guidelines and recipes, you'll enjoy delicious meals, snacks, and even desserts while giving your gut the nutrients it may lack. What's the result? A healthier gut and a happier you, no matter what your starting point is.

YOUR GUT, FROM THE INSIDE OUT:

DEBUNKING DIGESTIVE HEALTH MYTHS

When it comes to conditions like IBS, myths abound. "Oh, IBS is just a fancy name for gas and bloating." Or, "If you want to get rid of IBS, you should switch to a vegan diet." Or, "There's no way to reverse IBS."

I've heard them all! And I'm always amazed at the myths and misconceptions people— even those with medical backgrounds—have about IBS and other digestive disorders. One of the reasons I developed such a loyal following online is because I'm willing to uncover the truth behind the "facts" about IBS. I've been writing about this for years, but I'm still surprised at what people think is true when it comes to IBS and gut health in general.

But before we get into the myths, let's talk about how your gut functions. Then we'll unpack and debunk some of the biggest IBS and digestive health myths out there.

HOW YOUR DIGESTIVE SYSTEM WORKS

Have you ever thought about how amazing your digestive system is? It manages to take food—all different types of food, literally whatever you choose to eat—and extracts calories, or energy, and nutrients from it. Digestion actually starts in your mouth (which is why chewing your food properly is really important). Food then travels from there into your esophagus, into the stomach, then into the small intestine, the large intestine, and the anus. Your small intestine has three parts—the duodenum, the jejunum, and the ileum—and the large intestine includes your appendix, cecum, colon, and rectum. Your liver, pancreas, and gallbladder all also play a role in digestion.

The purpose of the digestive system is to break down the food you eat into pieces that are small enough for your body to absorb and use. Here's a closer look at what happens:

You take a bite of something. When you chew food, saliva helps begin to break down the starch in your food and starts the digestive process. When you swallow, the food travels through your esophagus into your stomach.

In your stomach, acid and enzymes break down the food, aided by stomach muscles that help mix the food with the digestive juices. Your pancreas sends digestive juice that includes enzymes that can break down protein, fats, and carbohydrates into your small intestine. Your liver joins the party, producing bile, a digestive juice that helps digest fats and certain vitamins. Your body's bile ducts transport the bile to the gallbladder until your gallbladder releases it while you're eating.

It's the small intestine that we're most interested in as far as IBS goes. Your small intestine makes its own digestive juice. It uses that digestive juice, along with the bile and digestive juice from the pancreas and enzymes produced by the bacteria that live in your gut, to continue breaking down and digesting the food. Your small intestine also absorbs water and other nutrients—in fact, it's responsible for most nutrient absorption (more about that in a bit!). Your circulatory system then steps up and sends them via your blood throughout your body; absorbed nutrients can cross the intestinal lining into your bloodstream. In the meantime, your liver stores some nutrients and can deliver them to your body later on.

In the large intestine, your GI tract sends more water back into your bloodstream, and the bacteria in your large intestine break down the remaining nutrients. Waste products and pieces of food that are still too large to be digested become stool.

People may not talk about the digestive process very often (unless they have trouble with it), but it's really an amazing system—when it works the way it's supposed to! But as you'll see in a minute, there are a number of things that can go wrong (and sadly do, even in people with healthy guts.)

Remember in the last chapter, when you learned that your gut and brain talk to each other? Different hormones and nerves are involved in your digestive process, and your brain and gut are in constant communication when it comes to the digestive process. Your stomach and small intestine are lined with

GUT BACTERIA: THE AMAZING MICROBIOME

There are billions (yup, that's right) of bacteria living in your intestines, especially in the large intestine and bowel. These bacteria, which are sometimes called gut flora or the microbiome, help with digestion. And your body needs to be able to digest all three kinds of macronutrients—protein, fat, and carbohydrates—as well as to digest and absorb the vitamins and minerals you get from food.

But these bacteria do more than just digest food; they are part of the immune system, and are constantly sending and receiving messages from the brain. While IBS isn't "in your head" as some might claim, there is definitely a connection between the brain and the gut. Researchers are continuing to study this fascinating link, but the biggest takeaway for me is that if you're anxious, upset, stressed out, or depressed, you're more likely to have GI symptoms. And, yes, just worrying about your GI symptoms can bring on more GI symptoms.

But remember, the opposite is true, too. When you learn how to eat and live in a way that makes you feel more confident and less worried about your ability to manage your IBS and GI symptoms, you may have fewer of them.

cells that create hormones that help control how much digestive juice is created, and they tell your brain whether you're hungry or full.

Your nerves play a role, too. For example, when you see or smell food that appeals to you, your brain lets your digestive system get ready to work. That's why your mouth may water or your stomach may growl. Other nerves located within your GI tract respond during the digestive process. Those nerves may signal that more digestive juice needs to be produced, or they may speed up or delay how fast food gets moved and pushed through your intestines.

You probably already know that you don't digest food well when you're upset or angry. You may be experiencing nerve interference. If you're out of alignment, nerves can get pinched, and when nerves get pinched or twisted, the signals from your brain that tell it to digest and contract may be compromised. That's one reason why chiropractic and therapeutic massages can help with good digestion.

Everyone suffers occasional stomach upset or digestive distress. That's normal and part of everyday life. What isn't, though, is when your gut is totally out of whack. In chapter 1, you learned about some of the factors that can make IBS worse. But what about what actually *causes* it? Researchers still don't know the cause of IBS, but I believe that some of the leading contenders are:

- **Gut dysbiosis.** You've just read about the gut bacteria, or the microbiome. Well, when your gut bacteria are out of balance,

your body can't digest and absorb food the way it's supposed to. Research shows that a lot of people with IBS have too few "good" bacteria and too many "bad" bacteria. We know that sometimes people get relief by consuming prebiotics (foods that feed the good bacteria) and probiotics (the good bacteria), but you can't just consume a ton of probiotics and call it a day. Still, though, gut dysbiosis is likely a big cause of common IBS symptoms, and my program will help you get that bacteria into a healthier balance.

- **Leaky gut.** Your GI tract is a long tube that is designed to keep the food and bacteria enclosed within it. Well, when your gut walls are damaged, little holes are created and your gut can "leak." This means that pieces of undigested food, bacteria, and other bad stuff can pass from your GI system into the rest of your body, and that causes inflammation and other symptoms. I could write a whole book about inflammation, but for our purposes, all you need to know is that it's how your body responds to perceived threats. It's bad for your overall health—chronic inflammation is linked to everything from a higher risk of heart disease and diabetes to many cancers and even obesity. But on the *Digest This* plan, you'll consume certain foods and supplements that help "heal and seal" your gut—including any damage you may have had already.

- **SIBO, or small intestinal bacteria overgrowth.** This happens when you simply have too many bacteria in your small intestine. The overgrowth of bacteria can damage your intestinal walls and trigger leaky gut syndrome, as well as cause IBS. I have had SIBO, but at the time I had no idea that was part of my problem. I thought I was experiencing a really bad IBS flare-up. SIBO symptoms are somewhat similar to many other IBS symptoms—things like gas, bloating, abdominal pain, and weight loss. However, if these symptoms just seem unbearable to the point you cannot even work or hold a job, and you're in the bathroom more than five times a day, SIBO may be something to look into in more depth.

- **Gut infections.** You saw in the last chapter that even one round of food poisoning increases your likelihood of having IBS by a factor of four. An infection in your gut isn't something like a cold, whereby your symptoms are obvious; instead, you may have one for months or years without realizing something is off, and in the meantime your gut health is going down the tubes.

- **Chronic dieting.** There isn't one person over the age of 15 who hasn't tried a diet of some sort. Heck, even my dad has gone on diets in the past! But when people diet, they often opt for low-calorie, low-carb, sugar-free, fat-free (and the list goes on)

WHAT YOU SHOULD KNOW ABOUT RESISTANT STARCH

While we're talking about prebiotics, let's cover a topic that is big news lately: resistant starch. Here's the deal. Most forms of starches are carbohydrates, but not all carbohydrates are created equal, and not all starches you consume get digested. Resistant starch is a type of carbohydrate that passes through your digestive tract unchanged. It can help lower blood sugar levels, improve insulin sensitivity, and is a prebiotic that can help improve your gut health.

Resistant starch passes through the stomach and small intestine undigested, reaching your colon, where it acts as food for the friendly bacteria in your gut to continue living and thriving. We all know that we need friendly bacteria in our guts to combat the bad bacteria; after all, bacteria (good or bad) are living organisms and need food, too! That's where resistant starch plays an important role.

chemical-filled diet foods. Manufacturers replace fat, carbs, and calories (a.k.a. energy) with chemicals that wreak havoc on your digestive system, kill off good gut bacteria, and mess with your microbiome. These changes can result in IBS.

THE BIGGEST MYTHS ABOUT IBS —AND THE FACTS BEHIND THEM

Now that we've covered some of the big contributing factors of IBS, let's switch gears and talk about some of the biggest myths about IBS—and the actual facts and truth behind them.

MYTH

IBS is all in your head.

FACT

Pretty much everyone I know who has dealt with a sick gut has heard this one. I'm here to tell you that sometimes you just have to ignore what people say. IBS is a real thing, whether or not you have a formal diagnosis of it. Surely 15 percent of the population aren't suffering from something that's "just in their heads."

But I know that some people just don't get it. My advice? Keep searching for answers and don't allow others' opinions to influence how you feel. After all, YOU are the only one who really can FEEL the way you do. Learn what you can about how to make your gut healthy and don't stop looking for answers (that's why you're reading this book, right?).

MYTH

A vegan diet (or any other overly restrictive diet) is the best diet to follow for IBS.

FACT

I've got nothing against vegans, and I understand that many people choose to follow vegan diets for health or ethical reasons. But a vegan diet didn't work for me. I tried it in an attempt to help my digestive issues at the time—but it didn't.

It was only when I started eating pureed animal protein and plain, whole-milk cultured Greek yogurt, along with other plant foods (and I do love fruits and veggies), that my gut began to heal. There's another issue here, too—if you rely on vegan versions of meats and cheeses, chances are you're consuming a lot of preservatives, chemicals, and—well—crap that is likely to make your gut problems even worse.

MYTH

Foods like protein bars and "superfood" green powders are good for you.

FACT

I've lost track of how many times I've blogged about this stuff, but let me break it down here. Most of the foods that are touted as being "healthy" are anything but. You can't be swayed by the claims or labels that manufacturers stick on their products. (And by the way, don't fall for labels that say "all natural." Rattlesnake venom is all natural, too, but that doesn't mean it's good for you!)

Let me make it super easy for you: Check the ingredients. That's the only way to know what's in the food you're eating. And when you see lots of weird names that you probably can't even pronounce, that's a sign that it's anything but healthy. In fact, a lot of these so-called healthy foods are loaded with additives like gums (you'll see words like "xanthan," "guar," and "locust bean") that are likely to make your digestive symptoms worse.

You probably already know that some ingredients like monosodium glutamate (MSG), the artificial sweetener Splenda, and carrageenan (an additive extracted from seaweed that can cause inflammation and bloating, and has been linked to cancer) are horrible for you. But there are a whole bunch of other ingredients that are still thought to be "healthy" and are marketed as such.

Some of the ingredients you want to avoid include:

- **Allulose.** This artificial sweetener is claimed to be "safe" and healthy, but there's controversy over its possible risks and side effects.

- **Brown rice syrup/rice syrup solids.** This common sweetener has a glycemic index of 98, which means it can send your blood sugar soaring. It's also often contaminated with arsenic, a poison.

- **Calcium chloride.** This is a common food additive that is also used to increase water hardness in swimming pools. Yuk!

- **Citric acid.** Also known as black mold. That's right—many food companies are now synthetically producing citric acid, a preservative, from black mold grown on food—and that's acceptable in the food industry!

- **Coconut milk powder.** You'd think this was a healthy choice, but to create a powder, food manufacturers use additives—so in other words, it's not just coconut milk powder! Skip it.

- **Erythritol.** This artificial sweetener is one of the worst additives you can consume if you have IBS—it's known to cause bloating and diarrhea.

- **Gums (like guar, locust bean, xanthan).** Gums are commonly used even in "health foods." They swell in the intestines, causing bloating, gas, cramping, and plenty of other issues.

- **Maltodextrin.** This additive is made when starchy plants—primarily corn—are broken down into monosaccharides using enzymes and, to a lesser extent, acids. Because it's from natural sources, dextrose is considered "natural," but it is still processed and can cause digestive upset.

- **Natural flavor/flavorings.** Here's the thing: "Orange" may be a natural flavor (because oranges are natural, right?), but that doesn't mean the flavoring in products came from natural sources.

- **Nutritional yeast.** Nutritional yeast is showing up in everything, and it's being pushed as a good source of B vitamins. I avoid this like the plague! In addition to digestive upset, it can cause yeast overgrowth and even skin rashes.

- **Peanuts/peanut butter.** Peanuts can become contaminated with a mold that produces aflatoxin, a known carcinogen associated with liver cancer. Any food that creates congestion in the liver may potentially impede its important functions, including detoxification.

- **Pork.** Organic or not, there's no escaping the issue that pigs are unable to release toxins because they have very few sweat glands. The result? You eat the toxins, too! In addition, pigs are common carriers of a variety of parasites—some that can't even be killed off when cooked.

MARISA'S STORY: WHEN WHAT YOU THINK IS HEALTHY . . . ISN'T

I became very ill about six years ago, and [then] three years ago it became chronic. Migraines, chronic headaches, fatigue, bloating, indigestion, and massive constipation. I was constipated for close to three months! I became so ill I [was] deeply depressed and missed out on life. [I dealt with] failed relationships, missing work, and not having a social life.

I randomly found you on Instagram, and WOW! I am so thankful. I started learning so much about my health, eating habits, and gut issues. One of the most important things I learned was how important it is to check ingredients! I immediately cut out maltodextrin and citric acid. Basically, everything "healthy" I was eating was not healthy at all! It took me about a year to get comfortable with my new habits. I will never look back! By changing my diet, I have healed my gut and found out the root cause of my chronic illness and pain.

—Marisa, 37

ANTIBIOTICS: BAD NEWS FOR YOUR GUT HEALTH

Here's the thing to remember about antibiotics. There are common bacterial infections—things like pneumonia, sinus infections, ear infections, strep throat, and acute bronchitis—that antibiotics may help treat because they kill the bacteria causing the infection. But if you have a cold or the flu, those are caused by a virus, not bacteria. And that means a round of antibiotics will do nothing—nothing—to help you get better.

I've been there, done that. I listened to my typical family practitioner years back and at least twenty times I took that Z-Pak they hand out like candy. You may already know that antibiotics kill the bad *and* the good bacteria in the body. But that's the least of your worries; you can replenish your body with good bacteria from high-quality cultured yogurt and probiotics. But antibiotics can do far more damage than that.

ANTIBIOTICS RAISE YOUR RISK OF DEVELOPING INFLAMMATORY BOWEL DISEASE

You know how antibiotics can sometimes get things moving down there a little faster than you'd like? That's because they're going to town on all kinds of bacteria—good and bad—totally disrupting the order of command in your intestines. While many see relief after stopping the antibiotic therapy, some people *never* recover, according to a 2011 study published in the *American Journal of Gastroenterology*. Researchers found that participants who took more than three antibiotics within a five-year period were one and a half times more likely to develop inflammatory bowel disease, or IBD. (While IBD is sometimes confused with IBS, the two conditions are different. Inflammatory bowel disease is the result of a malfunctioning immune system that causes inflammation and damage to the digestive system.)

ANTIBIOTICS MAKE YOU MORE LIKELY TO GAIN WEIGHT

You may already be aware that there are antibiotics in your meat (hence the fact that there are companies producing antibiotic-free protein). But did you ever wonder why farmers give animals antibiotics in the first place? Your first thought may be, "So I'm not eating a sick animal." Well, there are other ways to raise healthy animals without using antibiotics. So the question still stands: Why are antibiotics fed to animals?

They're used to fatten them up! (Scientists still aren't entirely sure why this works, but it does.) And they could be doing the same thing to your body. A 2015 study published in the *International Journal of Obesity* found that antibiotic use in childhood influences not only childhood weight gain but also weight gain *years later*. On a related note, antibiotics have also been linked to developing Type-2 diabetes—and obesity is a risk factor for diabetes.

ANTIBIOTICS MAY RAISE YOUR RISK OF DEPRESSION AND ANXIETY

We've talked about the gut-brain connection. Well, when antibiotics annihilate the bacteria in your gut—both the good and the bad—they're affecting your mind, too. According to a study published in 2015 in the *Journal of Clinical Psychology*, just a single course of antibiotics may be associated with a higher risk of depression and anxiety. And the risks can continue to rise with each subsequent antibiotic course. Researchers found that participants were 50 percent (yes, that's right—50 percent!) more likely to be diagnosed with depression or anxiety after five separate courses of penicillin. Luckily, I found out I was allergic to penicillin when I was young (I get severe hives all over my body) so that particular antibiotic was ruled out for me. However, penicillin is of course just one of many antibiotics doctors prescribe . . . and the list goes on and on.

I'm not telling you to refuse all antibiotics. They certainly have their uses, and I'm not your doctor. But I do want you to be aware of the risks and complications that can arise from taking them too freely.

- **Stevia.** How does a green leaf turn into a white powder you buy at the store? It goes through a 42-step process, and by the time it gets into your hands from the manufacturer, it's been altered and can cause tons of digestive issues, as well as headaches. It can also change your metabolism (and not for the better!), setting you up for weight gain.

- **Titanium dioxide.** Titanium dioxide, often found in many white vanilla cakes, salad dressings, coffee creamers, and chewing gum, may be a natural mineral found in the earth, but that doesn't make it healthy to consume. There are potential health concerns with this as a food ingredient, and I for one try to avoid it.

MYTH
You can cure your IBS with probiotics.

FACT

Probiotics can help you rebuild your gut health, but you should be aware that different probiotics may affect your gut differently.

Your best source of probiotics is high-quality cultured yogurt. That's one of the first foods I started eating when I created the *Digest This* plan, and I still eat at least 1 cup of it every day.

There are a ton of probiotics out there, but I recommend my Digestive Support Probiotic Nuzest Protein Powder (page 68) because it contains the probiotic *Bacillus coagulans*. This particular probiotic is one of the hardiest out there—it doesn't even need to be refrigerated and can withstand heat. It's also proven to be one of the most effective at fighting off candida and yeast overgrowth.

MYTH

Drinking kombucha can help your IBS symptoms.

FACT

Okay, I just talked about probiotics, but I get so many questions about kombucha in particular that it's worth talking about. I stay away from kombucha (unless it's homemade). The kind of kombucha you buy at the store can actually cause yeast overgrowth and SIBO from the sugars and cultures it contains. Many, if not all, companies use a probiotic strain called *Saccharomyces boulardii*, which can cause fungemia, the presence of fungi or yeasts in the bloodstream.

If you have a weak immune system, catch a cold easily, or suffer frequent yeast infections, you may be at higher risk for developing fungemia. Because many cultured food items like kombucha fail to indicate the type of probiotics they contain, you may be consuming *Saccharomyces boulardii* without realizing it. My advice? When in doubt, don't.

Even more important, the probiotics (regardless of the ones used) usually aren't even "alive" by the time they make it into the store. They go through many hands during the shipping process and by the time they get into stores and sit on the shelf for who knows how long, the living probiotics most likely are nonexistent. So you're basically paying for sugary, bubbly water.

And you know what? Kombucha can become addictive. I used to drink one a day (back in the days prior to my fungemia overgrowth), and it became quite expensive when I realized I "needed" my daily fix (oh, hey there, sugar!).

Yes, I know some people swear by their kombucha. To that I say two words: placebo effect. Plain and simple. I can't tell you not to drink it, but I can tell you why I choose not to. If you are prone to infections, or have IBS or digestion issues, you're better off avoiding it. Instead, try plain sparkling water (with no flavorings) and adding some juice, Vital Proteins beauty waters, powdered spirulina, and a squeeze of lemon.

By adding these ingredients and making your own flavors, you can mimic all the flavors out there commonly offered by kombucha brands—for a lot less money!

MYTH

Increasing fiber will help your IBS symptoms.

FACT

People with IBS-C, or IBS with constipation, are often told to eat more fiber to ease their constipation, but that can actually make your constipation worse. There are two types of fiber: soluble and insoluble. Soluble fiber blends well with water, forming a gel-like substance, whereas insoluble fiber does not blend well with water and acts as a "bulking agent" inside the gut to help move things along.

But what people fail to realize is that consuming too much fiber (especially in a short time period) will make things "bulk too much," so to speak, causing blockage and ultimately "stopping you up" even more so! Think about it, if a tube is clogged, would you want to add more bulk to that tube? Probably not! You would add liquid, oils, and lubricants to help break it up.

That's exactly what you need to do when you're constipated—and what you should do to continue to stay regular. If you're constipated, I always recommend that you do what I do: reduce your fiber intake and increase your liquids. (There are some fibers in certain fruits, like kiwi, that can help "get the job done.")

If you're constipated, I suggest drinking more fluids and consuming more avocado, eggs (with the yolks), and kiwifruits with the skins (that's where the valuable fiber is). Or consume a small amount of coconut oil (try 1 teaspoon and if that doesn't work, try up to 3 teaspoons throughout the day).

Things still aren't moving along? Try my bowel-moving drink, what I call the **Kicker Elixir:**

KICKER ELIXIR:

1 teaspoon cayenne

3 teaspoons ground cinnamon

1 teaspoon curry powder

1½ cups warm water

Optional: yacon syrup or unsulfured blackstrap molasses

Mix all the ingredients in a tall glass and consume it within 10 minutes. (You may start to feel warm from the spices.) Within 30 minutes, the drink should produce results.

MYTH

Your diet causes IBS. (Or consuming too many dairy products, or too much gluten, or too much anything causes IBS.)

FACT

This myth makes me crazy because it's that blame-the-victim thinking. It's like you did something that created your gut problems. Um, I don't think so!

Okay, yes, when you eat a lot of gut-irritating foods or crap that's full of chemicals and preservatives that your body can't digest, you're not doing your gut any favors. But your diet doesn't cause IBS.

I think it's important to recognize, though, that if you have food sensitivities or allergies, those can be confused with IBS, or may contribute to your digestive issues. If you're lactose-intolerant, for example, consuming dairy products can trigger similar symptoms. So, it

INULIN/CHICORY ROOT FIBER—GOOD OR BAD?

There's an ingredient that may be causing gas, bloating, severe cramping, and diarrhea—and yet it's something that you may be consuming *intentionally* to help with those issues! Say hello to chicory root fiber (sometimes also referred to as inulin or prebiotic fiber).

Yes, prebiotics are good for the gut, but bear with me. You may have seen "chicory root fiber" or "inulin" listed in the ingredients of your protein bar, protein powder, high-fiber cereals, breads, and even in your supplements. So what exactly is it?

Chicory root fiber is a special type of plant-based fiber. Like all fibers, it's indigestible by the human body. Inulin travels intact to the large intestine, where it contributes to the bulk of your stool, as well as acting as food for the friendly bacteria in your gut. Inulin naturally occurs in various produce and is commonly extracted from the roots of chicory plants and added to processed foods.

Prebiotics ARE good for the gut in their natural state (green banana, jicama, and artichokes are a few examples of prebiotics), but when they are extracted, broken down, manufactured, manipulated, and concentrated into a powder, this can cause some serious issues.

That is, when inulin is extracted and the prebiotic fiber is the only thing left, that's too much for your body to handle—even if it's put into a bar, cereal, or other food. It's now removed from its natural state and is now so concentrated it is causing more harm than good. Too much of a good thing is not a good thing!

Note, too, that the more fermenting your gut bacteria does, the more gas it produces. So large doses of prebiotic fibers like inulin can cause gastrointestinal distress. Individuals with IBS and digestive issues can experience symptoms at even minute doses. People with "normal" digestive function may be able to tolerate 10 grams of inulin without discomfort, but many foods contain 15 grams of this stuff in just one serving! And you may be eating multiple foods containing inulin every day, thinking it's benefiting you.

Another reason why inulin is added to many manufactured foods and snacks is so that they can claim "low carb" on the package. It's also cheap to manufacture. Adding fiber like inulin to foods bulks up and adds substance to the product, making it look bigger and keeping calories low per serving.

I personally stick to inulin in its natural state. If you want to incorporate prebiotic foods to help your friendly bacteria flourish, great! Just remember that you need only a little. Some natural sources of inulin include:

- Artichokes
- Asparagus
- Green/unripe bananas
- Jicama
- Leeks
- Onions

Note, too, that if you're allergic to ragweed, you should be careful about consuming inulin. It can also cause rare cases of "renal hypersensitivity." To avoid this, look for words like "inulin," "chicory root fiber," and "prebiotic fiber" on the labels of foods like:

- Energy, protein, meal-replacement, and granola bars
- Ready-to-drink protein shakes
- Low-calorie yogurts
- Low-calorie ice creams
- Non-dairy ice creams
- Non-dairy yogurts
- High-fiber "anything" (cereals, breads, bars)
- Gluten-free breads, waffles, bread/waffle mixes
- Digestive and herbal teas
- Probiotic supplements, powdered fiber supplements, or digestive health supplements

As I've said, each person is different. Chicory root fiber certainly upsets my gut, and I immediately experience the effects after consuming it, which is why I don't. If you have no problem with it, lucky you! But many people don't realize it's an ingredient that may be causing them issues in the first place.

My suggestion is to remove it from your diet for a week. After that week, buy something (like a bar), try it for yourself, and be mindful after eating it. See what happens and how you feel. That should be your confirmation right there!

can be hard to tease out what exactly the culprit is, and yes, your diet can aggravate your symptoms. But your diet does not *cause* IBS.

MYTH
IBS can't be reversed.

FACT

IBS can't be cured—that's the prevailing thought. And I would never say that I can cure anyone's IBS. But IBS can be reversed when you eliminate irritants and give your gut a chance to heal, to seal, and to re-create a healthy microbiome.

Does it happen overnight? Nope. But it can happen over days, weeks, or months. If I didn't believe that—and if I hadn't heard from thousands of people now who have seen it happen—I wouldn't be writing this book!

MYTH
Only women have IBS.

FACT

It's true that IBS strikes women more often than men, but men get it, too. Studies show that you're about two to two and a half times more likely to develop IBS if you're a woman, and women are also more likely to develop IBS after an infection.

Why are women more likely to get IBS? As it's more common among women in their mid-teens to mid-40s, it's likely that hormonal fluctuations play a role. (And as you saw in the last chapter, IBS may make premenstrual- and menstrual-related symptoms worse—and vice versa.) And women are far more likely to diet, and diet more frequently, than men, which also makes them more likely to develop digestive issues.

MYTH

IBS isn't that bad. It's just a little bit of gas and bloating.

FACT

Really? As you saw in chapter 1, for most people, IBS is more than a little gas and bloating. Symptoms may vary, but they're often debilitating enough for people to miss work (remember, the average person misses a day or two of work or school each month—and when you're in the midst of a flare-up, it may be far more than that). One of the reasons I'm so open about my symptoms and how I've struggled (but struggle much less now, thank goodness!) is that I know how isolating this condition can be.

MYTH

If you have IBS, you have to eat bland food the rest of your life.

FACT

I'm happy to say this myth is just that—a myth! Since my late teens, I've been into food. I love experimenting and creating healthy, delicious recipes that taste good and are good for your gut, too.

When I was at my worst (okay, let's face it—even today!), if I craved something, I was determined to make a healthy, easily digestible version of whatever that was. If I wanted bread, I made some. If I wanted a cookie or milkshake, I made a healthier option. Get creative! As you'll come to find throughout this book, there are no limits when it comes to developing healthier versions of classic recipes, even your favorites. And I'll show you how to do the same thing!

MYTH

IBS causes weight gain.

FACT

IBS affects different people in different ways. Yes, some people lose weight due to it, and some people's weight isn't affected. And some people do gain weight with IBS. It may be from hormonal imbalances, being unable to exercise, or feeling hungry and being unable to satisfy that hunger.

MYTH

IBS only affects digestion.

FACT

IBS can affect every aspect of your health. I always say, "It all starts in the gut" and your gut is your second brain. In fact, your gut is the center and "home" to so many other areas in your body. Think of it as the root, and all areas of your body are connected and branch out from the center.

That means that when your gut is unhealthy, it impacts other aspects of your health, too—things like your skin, hair, and brain, not to mention your mental health! As you learned earlier, if you have IBS, you're more likely to suffer from depression and anxiety. Digestive problems can even affect your hormones, which in turn can affect everything from your menstrual cycle to your sex drive to the quality of your sleep, your hair, your mood, and even your hunger levels. Heck, I experienced it all!

Your outside appearance really does come from within, and when your gut is malfunctioning, you simply can't look your best, either. You can't change your genetics—they determine, for example, the texture of your hair. I for one always had super-thin, baby-fine hair and both of my parents suffered from severe acne, so I was likely to get it, too.

But the health of my skin and hair suffered, in part because of IBS, and my brain function suffered as well. It was difficult for me to think straight. I had a hard time concentrating, and I would lash out at my parents for no reason at all. On top of all that, I struggled with depression, and that was made even worse when I missed out on events and was unable to socialize—while I saw friends going out, having fun, getting married, and

living their lives. That was really hard for me. In retrospect, I know this exacerbated my symptoms. It was a hard pattern to break out of, but I did—and you can, too!

MYTH

Changing your diet is the only way to treat IBS.

FACT

Yes, diet matters, but there are other strategies that work, too. For example, CBD (cannabidiol; see sidebar, page 46) is becoming one of the latest ways to help treat IBS. In addition to stress management (which we'll talk about in the next chapter), we now know that there is interplay between nerve function and gut health. Think of it this way: If your nerves are pinched, they may not be able to send the signals between the gut and brain; and if those signals don't get through, there's a disconnect.

What this means is that things like chiropractic care, nerve stimulation, meditation, and other "nontraditional" techniques may help improve your digestive health. We'll talk more about them in the next chapter.

MYTH

The FODMAP is the best diet to treat IBS.

FACT

The FODMAP diet (see chapter 1) may be the suggested diet for people with IBS, but all it

CAN CBD HELP WITH IBS?

CBD is the latest thing—chances are, you know someone who's using it or maybe you've tried it yourself. It turns out it may be helpful for IBS, as well.

CBD is the abbreviation for cannabidiol, the primary non-psychoactive component of the plant *Cannabis sativa* (marijuana). Many people confuse it with THC (tetrahydrocannabinol), the component in marijuana that does have psychoactive effects and is what makes people "high"—but the two are different.

Both do have health benefits—THC has antispasmodic, analgesic, anti-tremor, and anti-inflammatory properties, and can stimulate the appetite (hence, the "munchies"). CBD also has anti-inflammatory benefits and anticonvulsant, antipsychotic, and neuro-protective properties, which means it helps your nervous system function properly. It also has pain-relieving properties and helps reduce anxiety.

According to a recent paper published in the journal *Cannabis and Cannabinoid Research*, cannabis has been used for ages to treat a variety of gastrointestinal disorders. Simply put, CBD may help improve gastrointestinal function and gut motility, support healthy gut microbiota, and help heal leaky gut syndrome.

Remember that the gut is lined with epithelial cells that are linked together by tight junction proteins. These tight junctions act like barriers between your gut and your bloodstream, keeping the "good stuff" in your bloodstream and the "bad stuff" out.

In cases of leaky gut, the tight junctions become increasingly porous and allow access to the bloodstream by harmful bacteria and pathogens. Your gut plays an essential role in your immune system and when you have leaky gut, you're more likely to get sick more easily, catching anything and everything that comes your way. Chronic stress, poor diet, and an imbalance in the gut microbiome can all cause leaky gut. Scary, huh?

Well, the good news is that CBD may be the answer to decreasing the permeability at tight junctions. Recent research found that CBD has been shown to directly restore endothelial membrane permeability—in other words, make your gut less leaky!

And I know firsthand that CBD can help. I started taking CBD in 2017 because it's known to relax the intestinal muscles, as well as block gastrointestinal mechanisms that produce stomach pain associated with IBS. Studies show that CBD helps reduce spontaneous intestinal movements and alleviates both colonic spasms and abdominal pain, as well as nerve pain.

The bottom line? CBD may be worth trying for IBS. Keep in mind, though, that everyone's experience is different. Start with a relatively low dosage. Note, too, that because CBD can relax the intestines and muscles, it also relaxes the mind and may make you sleepy (it does for me!). So, it may be best to take it at night (at least at first).

THE IMPORTANCE OF SLEEP

IBS affects every aspect of your life, including sleep. If you have IBS or gut health issues, you're also more likely to have insomnia and other sleep problems. Not surprising, right?

But did you know that our bodies can (and do) withstand years of poor nutrition, but if you go more than eleven days without sleep, you can die? It's true. Sleep deprivation is so damaging to the body that it's been used as a form of torture!

We spend so much time, money, and energy on our diets and workout routines yet we often forget or ignore the quality and quantity of our sleep. How can you expect your body to perform, grow, repair, heal, and ultimately be healthy without enough sleep? In short, you can't deprive yourself of sleep and then expect it to perform miracles during the day.

Eight to nine hours of sleep is optimal for most adults, but some people actually need more depending on what's happening in their lives. If you're under a lot of stress, training hard, even juggling more than usual, you may need more sleep. New research suggests that sleep problems may trigger IBS symptoms or make them worse, so getting quality sleep should be part of your overall lifestyle when you're working on healing your gut. Another bonus? You're more likely to maintain a healthy body weight, age more slowly, and maintain clear skin when you get enough sleep!

does is eliminate certain carbohydrates from your diet. First off, not all those carbohydrates may irritate your specific gut. Second, it ignores other irritants that may play a bigger role. But most important, the FODMAP diet only seeks to avoid gut irritation. It doesn't tell you what to eat to help heal and seal your gut.

What should you eat? Foods like papaya, pineapple, mango, and kiwi all contain essential digestive enzymes that should be consumed on a regular basis. (Don't worry—you'll learn much more about these foods and find plenty of recipes that include them in the following chapters, including my Digestive Boost [page 101], a drink that contains fruits with specific enzymes to help regulate your digestion.)

Now that you have your facts straight about IBS and how your gut is meant to function, you're ready to learn more about the *Digest This* plan, including the Gut Reset. This unique program is based on foods that will help heal your gut in just three weeks—and may have you noticing a dramatic change in your gut function in even less time than that.

So, let's get started!

21 DAYS TO A HEALTHY GUT:

THE GUT RESET

Before we jump into basics of the Gut Reset, let me tell you how I developed it and the *Digest This* plan. I suffered from IBS for years, and by the time I was in my mid-20s, I realized that doctors and conventional treatments had failed me. The only person who had ever been able to help me was a holistic doctor I'd seen as a teen.

After talking with him, I decided to make some radical diet changes. I started experimenting with what worked for me—and what didn't. I eliminated gut-irritating foods, cut out foods that were hard to digest (like raw vegetables), reduced my intake of carbs, and started eating a diet high in organic chicken and grass-fed beef. I needed the nutrients! I pureed my pre-cooked chicken and beef to make it easier to digest (don't worry—it's better tasting than you might think!), and started consuming bone broth, collagen, and gelatin to help heal my damaged gut.

And amazingly, I started to feel better in a few weeks. I paid close attention to what worked for my body and what didn't. I educated myself about digestive health and the impact that things like additives, gums, and everyday ingredients can have on the digestive system. I continued to follow an all-soft, mostly pureed diet for several months, and my IBS symptoms disappeared. Gone were the pain, the bloating, and the sudden trips to the bathroom. I regained the weight my body needed and was able to lead a normal life—one I thought was unattainable.

THE GUT RESET PROGRAM WAS BORN

In doing this, I realized that I'd developed a program to treat IBS—a program that people desperately needed. I started sharing the principles of the program with my followers in 2016. Since then, thousands of followers have taken my advice and healed their guts—and improved the quality of their lives, as well. I've taken their crowd-testing and experiences into account as I've continued to fine-tune the elements of the program. I've also continued to notice (good) changes in my body years after healing, and I'm happy to report that it just keeps getting better!

You may be in pain. You may be miserable. You may have given up hope. I had! And you can't wait for researchers, scientists, and physicians to figure out what they *think* the best plan to treat IBS is—and the fact is, there may never be agreement on it! *You* need a program you can try today, knowing that you'll be feeling better in a matter of weeks, maybe even days. That's what my program will help you do.

When your gut is in crisis, radical action is necessary. And that's where my 21-day Gut Reset comes in. I won't candy-coat it for you. This is an intense, strict, radical way of eating—and it will be challenging to stick with it. It's gonna be tough. You may look at the principles and think, *That's all I get to eat? How will I survive?*

If that's you, then ask yourself how lousy you feel. How miserable you are with symptoms you can't control—or can't control for longer than a few days. How tired you are of having your life on hold. Now, are you willing to spend just 21 days to help heal and reset your gut—and then spend the weeks, months, and years after that feeding it with the foods that it needs so that it can function optimally? I bet you are.

Besides, my plan is super simple, and it works.

After the Gut Reset, you're free to step outside the strictures of the program and include other foods in your diet during the maintenance period. My *Digest This* plan is divided into these two parts because many—but not all—people need a radical intervention to start the healing process. If your symptoms aren't that bad, you may find it difficult to stay on the Gut Reset for the three weeks, and quite frankly, you may not need to. (I hope you consider it, though—your gut can do a *lot* of healing when you provide it with the Gut Reset foods in this relatively short time period!)

During the second part of the *Digest This* plan—you know, the rest of your life—you continue to avoid gut irritants and you *should* continue to follow the Gut Reset principles, especially the last two. I want you to pick and choose what works for you—this is your life, and I want you to have freedom, not fear, when it comes to food. Just keep in mind that the longer you've had digestive issues, the longer it will take to repair the damage.

Why make the effort? Because it will pay off. In just three weeks, you'll have started the process of healing your gut and can begin to feed it delicious foods you may have thought were off-limits—all the while continuing to live symptom-free. You'll then be free to enjoy the rest of the recipes in the rest of this book, and to adapt and modify them as you like. You'll be able to enjoy food again. To be free from pain, digestive issues, and the fear, anxiety, and dread you may have been suffering for years. With a healthy gut, you're free to not just **survive** from day to day but also to **thrive.**

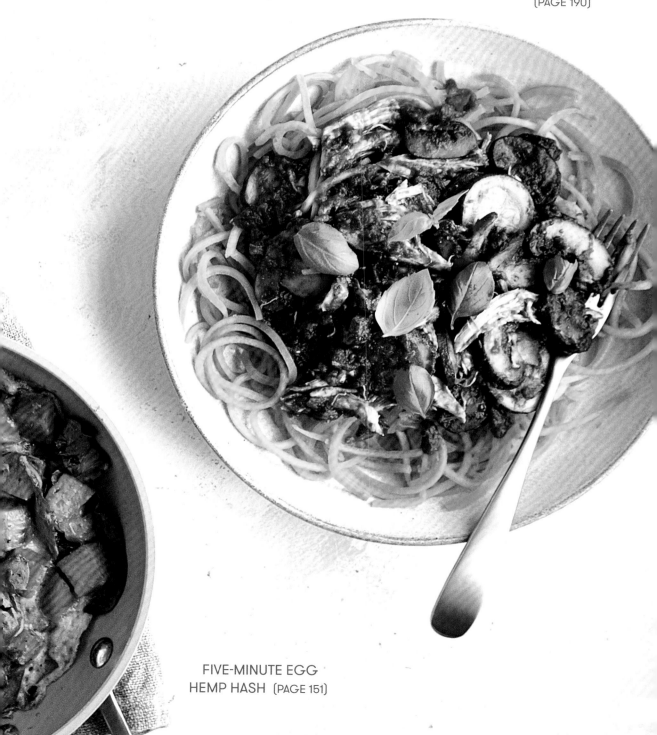

GRAIN-FREE
BUTTERNUT PASTA
(PAGE 190)

FIVE-MINUTE EGG
HEMP HASH (PAGE 151)

THE GUT RESET: 21 DAYS TO A HEALTHIER GUT— AND A HEALTHIER YOU

Let's talk about the basics of eating with IBS. Forget the basic four food groups or the food pyramid. If you have gut issues like IBS, you should divide foods into three different groups:

- **Gut irritants.** These foods (like raw veggies, beans, sugar, stevia, and wheat) tend to irritate the gut and should be avoided.

- **Gut-neutral foods, or "gut neutrals."** These foods (like avocados, chicken, nut butters, and rice) tend to have more of a neutral impact, neither healing nor irritating your gut.

- **Gut-healing foods, or "gut healers."** These foods actually help heal and rebuild the gut. They include foods like plain, whole-milk cultured Greek yogurt and bone broth, and they are the backbone of the 21-day Gut Reset and the *Digest This* plan.

Here you'll find more comprehensive lists of each:

GUT IRRITANTS

- Alcohol
- Allulose, a sweetener
- Berries (especially raspberries and blackberries)
- Brown rice syrup/rice syrup solids
- Calcium chloride, a food additive
- Cheese (unless goat or sheep)
- Chicory root fiber (a.k.a. inulin), a common additive
- Citric acid, a food additive
- Coconut milk powder
- Corn (whole kernels and popped; if it's ground into a flour, it is okay)
- Dextrose/cultured dextrose (artificial sugar)
- Erythritol, a sugar alcohol used as a sweetener
- Figs
- Gluten (except cultured, such as in sourdough bread)
- Gums (guar, xanthan, locust bean, etc.), common additives
- Kombucha
- Letiticin (soy and sunflower), a type of oil
- Maltodextrin, a common additive
- Milk (but cultured yogurt, kefir, and goat milk are okay)
- Natural flavor and flavorings
- Nutritional yeast
- Peanuts, peanut butter
- Pork
- Soy products
- Stevia
- Titanium dioxide, a food coloring

- Vitamin A palmitate, an additive used to replace fat
- Wheat and wheat bran
- Whole, small seeds like chia, sesame, and flax (unless ground into a paste or in a smoothie)
- Yeast extract

In addition to these Gut Irritants, other foods can be irritating to many guts, but some people can tolerate them in small amounts. They include:

- Almonds (with their skins on)
- Artichokes
- Asparagus
- Beets
- Cayenne
- Celery
- Coconut water
- Dried or dehydrated fruit
- Garlic
- Grapefruits
- Grapes
- Kale
- Kimchi
- Melon
- Mushrooms
- Nightshades (like white potatoes and eggplant)
- Nutmeg
- Onion
- Oranges
- Peppers
- Radishes
- Tomatoes
- Watermelon

GUT NEUTRALS

- Apples
- Avocados
- Bananas
- Beef
- Carrots (cooked)
- Cauliflower
- Cherries
- Chicken
- Chickpeas (garbanzo beans)
- Coconut
- Coffee
- Cucumbers (with skins removed)
- Dates
- Eggs
- Fish
- Golden potatoes
- Green beans (cooked)
- Kidney beans
- Nut and seed butters (smooth, not chunky)
- Olives
- Pears
- Peas
- Persimmons
- Rice
- Sourdough bread
- Spinach (in small amounts)
- Sprouted rolled oats
- Sweet potatoes
- Turkey
- Wild blueberries
- Winter squash (acorn, butternut, kabocha, pumpkin)
- Zucchini

GUT HEALERS

- Bone broth
- Chamomile tea
- Cultured Greek yogurt (full-fat, plain)
- Cultured kefir
- Ginger
- Kiwi
- Lemon
- Mango
- Olive leaf tea
- Papaya
- Pineapple
- Peppermint
- Unsweetened chocolate or cacao

In addition, these supplements that can be taken in powder or oil form are very healing to the gut:

- CBD (see sidebar, page 46)
- Collagen
- Gelatin
- L-glutamine
- Pea protein

It should be clear that you need both a healthy gut—to digest and absorb the nutrients in food—and a diet that is nutritious and irritant-free for optimal gut health. It's actually *better* to have good digestion with a bad diet than bad digestion and a good diet; with the former, at least you can absorb *something*. But there's no point in consuming nutritious foods if you can't absorb them, right? That's what is so awesome about my plan. By simply consuming the right foods and avoiding the destructive ones, you'll be both consuming the nutrients your body needs and improving your gut's ability to completely digest them!

So, let's take a closer look at the eight principles of the program, and then we'll look at each element in more depth:

- **Principle #1:** Eat pureed animal protein every day.

- **Principle #2:** Eat plain, whole-milk cultured Greek yogurt (preferably with rice) every day.

- **Principle #3:** Consume the Digestive Boost (page 101), a fruit enzyme drink, every morning.

- **Principle #4:** Consume bone broth every day.

- **Principle #5:** Consume only foods that are included in the Gut Reset program.

- **Principle #6:** Take gelatin, collagen, and/or L-glutamine every day (often in the form of smoothies).

- **Principle #7:** Turn on the parasympathetic nervous system before you eat. (You may not think this is important but it's crucial.)

- **Principle #8:** Perform at least one stress-reduction technique every day.

PRINCIPLE #1:
EAT PUREED PROTEIN (FREE-RANGE CHICKEN OR GRASS-FED BEEF) EVERY DAY

I made this the first principle because it's that important. During the 21 days of the Gut Reset, you'll do something you've probably never done before. You'll puree your protein, and you'll consume plenty of pureed protein every day.

I want you to choose the healthiest protein options you can. Preferably that means grass-fed organic beef or pasture-raised organic chicken or turkey. All are free from hormones, antibiotics, and other crap that can interfere with your gut.

Then I want you to puree it, which makes it much easier for your body to digest and absorb in this severe state. (Remember that the first step of the digestive process is chewing your food, which helps break it down into smaller pieces.) Well, because your protein is pureed, you don't have to chew it—it's predigested, and has the consistency of hummus.

Pureeing the protein also makes it incredibly nutrient-dense and compact; ½ cup of pureed organic chicken, for example, is the equivalent of eating an entire three-ounce chicken breast. You'll be able to consume the nutrients your body needs without experiencing bloating or feeling over-full.

PRINCIPLE #2:
EAT PLAIN WHOLE-MILK CULTURED GREEK YOGURT EVERY DAY

In chapter 2, you learned about the microbiome, or gut flora, that is essential to healthy, normal digestion. Your gut needs the right balance of good bacteria, called probiotics, to function optimally. While you can buy probiotic supplements, I'm not a fan of them for several reasons, as discussed in the previous chapter. In fact, taking too many probiotics in the form of pills and powder can actually do more harm than good—even the "good" bacteria wind up fighting each other and offset the benefit of taking them.

I prefer that you get your probiotics from food—in this case, from plain, whole-milk cultured Greek yogurt. (You can choose plain, whole-milk cultured regular yogurt if you like, but because it has been strained of liquid, Greek yogurt has more concentrated protein than regular yogurt.) The probiotics found in the plain yogurt (which contains no added sugar or other ingredients) help to build up the healthy bacteria and reset your microbiome—gently and without reliance on probiotics.

Ideally you'll eat your yogurt with some plain cooked white or brown rice—your choice. The rice is a prebiotic, or a food that feeds the probiotics. Cool, huh?

PRINCIPLE #3:
CONSUME A DIGESTIVE BOOST EVERY MORNING

Beyond gut-healing foods like Greek yogurt and bone broth, certain foods contain digestive enzymes that help break down food. The right combination of these enzymes helps boost your gut's ability to break down, absorb, and mobilize food easily through your system.

My Digestive Boost (page 101) consists of kiwi, mango, papaya, and pineapple. Each food is rich in different digestive enzymes, and they all have other positive health impacts, as well. Plan on drinking it the first thing in the morning, or with breakfast or your mid-morning snack. Let's look at each of them in turn.

Kiwi: Kiwi is a digestive dynamo! It contains an enzyme called actinidin, which helps your body break down the protein found in meat, dairy foods, eggs, and fish, as well as in non-animal sources of protein like legumes and cereals. Research has found that consuming more of this enzyme helps improve your body's ability to digest protein more fully—what researchers call "enhancing the gastric hydrolysis proteins" in food.

Mango: Mangoes contain digestive enzymes called amylases. Amylases break down complex carbohydrates into "simple" sugars like glucose and maltose, which are easier for your body to absorb and use. (Your pancreas and salivary glands also produce amylase enzymes, but mangoes help make sure that you're getting enough of them.) The riper a mango is, the more active the amylase enzymes are, so look for ripe mangoes for your Digestive Boost.

Papaya: Did you know that papaya is often used as a meat tenderizer? That's because it contains an enzyme called papain, which helps break down protein. Ripe, uncooked papaya has been associated with the reduction of IBS symptoms like constipation, bloating, and heartburn.

Pineapple: Pineapple is the only major food source of the enzyme bromelain. It's concentrated within the core but is found throughout the fruit. This enzyme helps break down protein, and also has been proven to reduce inflammation, suppress cancer cells, and speed recovery from surgery by reducing bruising, swelling, and pain.

PRINCIPLE #4:
CONSUME BONE BROTH EVERY DAY

Bone broth is made from the bones and ligaments of animals that have been simmered for a long time; it's jam-packed with nutrients that will also help rebuild your gut. Studies show that bone broth is beneficial for restoring the strength of the gut lining and fighting food sensitivities (like wheat or dairy), helping with the growth of probiotics (good bacteria) in the gut, and decreasing inflammation levels in the digestive tract.

Studies have also found that people with digestive imbalances have lower levels of collagen (the protein that gives structure to connective tissue, including bones, ligaments, tendons, and, yes, the walls of your digestive tract) in their blood. Because the amino acids in collagen build the tissue that lines the entire GI tract, supplementing with collagen can improve digestion and treat leaky gut syndrome. And it helps improve joint health, boost immune function, and maintain healthy skin, as well.

Look for bone broth that has been made from pasture-raised or grass-fed animals and is very low in sodium.

PRINCIPLE #5:
CONSUME ONLY FOODS THAT ARE INCLUDED IN THE GUT RESET PROGRAM

This principle is simple but very important. My plan eliminates foods with preservatives, artificial ingredients, and other additives that can quite literally make you sick. The idea of the Gut Reset is that you're going to consume only Gut Neutrals and Gut Healers. But don't worry. All of the Gut Reset foods and smoothies provide you with the additional nutrients that your gut needs to heal, and they're completely free from all gut irritants.

PRINCIPLE #6:
TAKE GELATIN, COLLAGEN, OR L-GLUTAMINE EVERY DAY

I'm not a big fan of supplements; I prefer to get my nutrients from food. This, however, is where I make an exception. Gelatin is high in protein and helps heal and rebuild the gut, sealing any holes that have been created. Gelatin helps keep the good stuff in your digestive tract (and the bad stuff out!), and prevents undigested food from leaking into the bloodstream, which triggers inflammation. Gelatin also supports skin, nail, and hair growth; enhances joint health; and even helps tighten loose skin and improve the appearance of cellulite.

You've already learned a little bit about collagen, which is found in bone broth. I recommend you take additional collagen to make sure you're getting enough. It comes in powder form and it's super easy (and fun!) to get creative with how you use it. You can add collagen powder to pretty much anything—sweet, savory, baked, cooked, you name it. Heck, you can even add it to plain old water and won't taste it! I use and recommend Vital Proteins collagen and gelatin, and you'll find them as an ingredient in many of the smoothies later in the book, as well as in other recipes.

L-glutamine is an essential amino acid—a building block of protein that our bodies can't make, and is used to repair and rebuild the digestive tract. This amino acid is often taken by athletes to promote muscle recovery, but I've personally found it extremely helpful for my gut, possibly because the digestive tract is full of muscle that contracts and releases to help digest food and move it along. L-glutamine also promotes brain health, which may have a corresponding impact on gut health, as we understand more about the link between the gut and the brain. L-glutamine also appears to help normalize your gut's mucus production, as well as curb cravings for sugar and alcohol. (Look for a brand that has L-glutamine as the only ingredient on the label.)

PRINCIPLE #7:
TURN ON THE PARASYMPA-THETIC NERVOUS SYSTEM BEFORE YOU EAT

So far we've been talking about what you eat. Now I want you to think about *how* you eat. Be honest: How often do you eat while doing something else, like working or texting or keeping up with Instagram (um, guilty?). If the answer is "all the time," let me tell you that you're not doing your digestive system any favors.

Here's why. Your body's autonomic nervous system is responsible for involuntary reactions and responses to information your body receives. Your sympathetic nervous system is called into action when your brain determines that there is a threat; the "fight or flight" response is then triggered. Your heart rate and breathing rate increase. Your blood pressure rises. Blood is shunted away from your internal organs to your extremities to prepare your body to fight off an attacker or to run away to safety.

The parasympathetic nervous system, on the other hand, triggers a state of calm. The opposite of "fight or flight," it's called the "rest and digest" response. When this system is triggered, your blood pressure, heart rate, and respiration drop. Blood is shunted to your internal organs, including your digestive system, to enable them to do the important work of digesting and absorbing the food you eat, and sending those nutrients throughout your

body. When your parasympathetic system is turned on, you feel relaxed. Calm. At peace.

Simple enough, right? Well, here's the problem. Our bodies are designed to have these two systems work together. After the sympathetic nervous system fires up, the parasympathetic system should switch "on" and bring your body back to equilibrium. However, that's not what happens to most of us in our day-to-day lives.

There are two problems. First off, our bodies interpret things as potential dangers that may not actually be dangers. So, your body's "fight or flight" response is continually being triggered. Second, most of us (including me!) have a hard time getting that stress response under control. (That's where the eighth principle of the *Digest This* plan comes in.)

Your parasympathetic system is the "rest and digest" system that helps lower stress hormones like cortisol and adrenaline, and improves digestive function. So, it makes sense that you want to turn on the parasympathetic system before you eat.

How do you flip that switch? By interrupting your busy day with activities that turn it on. That might mean taking a short walk outside, reading something for pleasure (nothing too stimulating!), or a couple of minutes of slow, deep breathing. I might read my Bible, take a hot shower, watch a funny YouTube video, or call a friend to chat. These things help me flip the switch, so you'll want to figure out how to flip yours.

PRINCIPLE #8:
PERFORM AT LEAST ONE STRESS REDUCTION TECHNIQUE EVERY DAY

The idea behind turning on the parasympathetic system before you eat is simple: to activate the "rest and digest" system that fosters calm and, not coincidentally, better digestion. And that's great in the short term. But I want you to take a longer-term approach as part of the 21-day Gut Reset. I want you to start getting a handle on stress—the everyday stress you probably don't even think about anymore—and manage it better.

First off, this is simply better for your overall health. Even low-level stress, when it's constant, makes you more likely to develop everything from heart disease to diabetes to high blood pressure to many kinds of cancer. It also means you're more likely to suffer from depression and anxiety. But since we're focusing on IBS and digestive health here, let's consider one aspect of stress reduction: You'll improve your gut health.

I know, you may be rolling your eyes at this ("But I don't have time to manage my stress!"). Or maybe you're thinking, *I'm not really that stressed*. But if you have IBS, or digestive issues, you're almost certainly stressed. The problem is that often we get so used to being stressed that it becomes our new normal—even when it's anything but.

One of the trickiest aspects of managing stress is figuring out what stresses you

SIGNS OF OVER-EXERCISE

Yes, exercise is good for your body, and your digestive health. But too much of it can have the opposite effect. Signs that you're over-exercising include:

- Being unable to perform well or make additional gains at the gym ("plateauing")
- Loss of enjoyment in exercise
- Constantly feeling tired or fatigued
- Feeling depressed or sad
- Mood swings, irritability, or feeling angry for no reason
- Trouble sleeping
- Feeling extremely sore after workouts
- Getting sick frequently
- Feeling anxious or out of sorts
- Having trouble digesting food
- Feeling bloated or like food is "stuck"

If you notice these kinds of symptoms, give your body a break by taking some time (two or three days, to up to a week) off from working out. If they're caused by over-exercise, they should dissipate fairly quickly.

out—and what helps you handle it. Everyone is different! I spend pretty much all day, almost every day, on social media. I love it. I love sharing my recipes and research with my followers, and I love staying connected with people. It's my passion! But I know the idea of being on social media the way I am would make other people bonkers.

The same goes for exercise. I find exercise a great way to de-stress. I love the feeling of going to the gym, of doing a hard workout, of challenging my body. It's tiring, but it's also energizing to me.

But too much exercise isn't good for you, either! If I work out too much or for too long (45 minutes is plenty for one day), I can do more damage than good to my digestive system. I used to think "more is more" when it came to exercise, but as I've personally realized—along with research and feedback from my followers—sometimes the best thing we can do is *rest*. In fact, I consciously choose to take an exercise break every few weeks to give my body and mind a break.

Hey, for many of us, it's hard not to work out. I get it. It lifts our moods and gets those endorphins flowing. But exercise can sometimes interfere with your digestion, because it puts your body into that sympathetic state. Your heart rate is up, you're breathing faster, and the blood is flowing to your working muscles. That's great and helps get you fitter, but sometimes it's hard to get your body back into that parasympathetic state. Hard or extended workouts make it even more difficult. You want to wait at least an hour after a workout to let your body settle back into a parasympathetic state before you sit down to eat.

So, what are some of the best ways to de-stress? Effective techniques include:

- Exercise—in the right amount
- Meditation (learn how to do this in the next chapter!)
- Keeping a gratitude journal
- Prayer
- Connection; call a friend—even a quick check-in text can help
- Read
- See a movie—even by yourself!
- Try a new hobby (like ceramics, drawing, knitting, photography)
- Clean your place (that may seem like a chore but when my house is clean, I feel less stressed!)
- De-clutter your home; donate items you don't wear, need, or use (You'll feel better having less. I do!)

Because the brain-gut connection plays a factor in IBS, managing the stress you feel on a daily basis can have a powerful impact on your overall digestive health.

* * *

THAT'S IT! Now that you know all the elements of the 21-day Gut Reset program, you'll learn how to prepare for it in the next chapter. And don't worry—in just three short weeks, you'll have access to the delicious, simple recipes that will help keep your newly healed gut functioning at its best.

GET SET FOR THE 21-DAY GUT RESET

How are you feeling? Now that you've learned the basics of the *Digest This* plan, it's time to take a deep breath—then dive in. You're about to embark on a three-week adventure of changing (possibly radically changing) the way you eat.

No, it won't be easy. But I promise it will be worth it.

Remember: Everything you eat can be lumped into three basic categories—Gut Irritants, Gut Neutrals, and Gut Healers. The idea of the Gut Reset is to completely eliminate all irritants and then to heal, seal, and rebuild your gut from the inside out (literally) with the healing foods your gut is begging for.

GEARING UP FOR SUCCESS

However, just as you wouldn't go on a long vacation without making some plans ahead of time (packing list, anyone?), I don't expect you to jump right into this program without preparing ahead of time. So, let's break down your prepping into three basic phases:

- Having the right attitude

- Having the right tools

- Having the right foods

THE RIGHT ATTITUDE

I know this is a book about IBS, so you might think that I'd start off by talking about what you're going to be eating (and not eating!). Well, guess again. I want to start by suggesting that you begin by making sure you have the right attitude going into this program. And that means a couple of things.

First, it means committing to the program. I don't know how miserable you are right now, but the worse you feel, the more motivated you may be. And that's great! But what happens a few days in, when you start feeling better, and you think, well, one doughnut/piece of pizza/hunk of cheese/fill-in-the-blank won't hurt that much—and then you end up undoing the healing that your body has started.

Or maybe you're not feeling *that* sick, at least not right now, and you don't know if sticking to the Gut Reset for three weeks (*three whole weeks?! Really?*) is worth it.

I'm not here to tell you how to live your life, though I am here to help you, if you'll let me. So, let me say it like this: *It all comes down to* you, and your choices. No, you may not be able to help having IBS, and you may not even know why you developed it. But you can help yourself, starting today, with the choices you make. And I promise you, if you follow this plan, and eat only Gut Neutrals and Gut Healers (and avoid the Gut Irritants!), your gut will heal.

Your gut may not be 100 percent healthy at the end of three weeks, but you'll be well on your way to a healthier gut, more radiant skin, better mood, higher energy level—you name it. And you'll notice these kinds of changes in just a matter of days.

Sometimes eliminating foods from your diet may not seem beneficial, or you may not notice a dramatic effect right away. But if you avoid them for several weeks, and then try reintroducing them, you'll know if you're sensitive to them.

Take stevia, for example. When I decided to eliminate stevia from my diet, I honestly wondered if it was necessary and whether it would make a difference. Three weeks went by, I was feeling great, so I thought, *Hmmm, I'm feeling fine so why should I eliminate this?* And within five minutes of having some stevia, I had a horrible headache and I was bloated like a balloon! I never really knew how much it affected me (along with other foods and ingredients) until I tried it after first eliminating it.

This may not be the case for you and you may in fact feel a difference immediately after removing gut-irritating foods and additives. However, it takes a while for your body to rid itself of irritants. If you avoid

AVA'S STORY: LEARNING HOW TO QUESTION WHAT YOU PUT IN YOUR BODY

I've basically had digestive issues all my life. I've always had a super-slow system, and because of it I've dealt with acid reflux, constipation, bloating, and gas.

My symptoms made it really hard for me to go out, because my stomach would always feel full and achy and gassy. Eating often resulted in stabbing stomach pains. I've struggled since I was ten, so all the doctor recommended that I do was laxatives and MiraLAX. It helped with the constipation, but I always felt so awful.

After finding you on Instagram, I was just beginning my own health journey. I was starting to eat "healthier," but it wasn't until I found you that my definition of health became much more real. I learned to read ingredients and question what I was putting in my body being recommended by "health" influencers. I avoid gums and fillers at all costs, and I'm not trying to consume a ton of raw veggies and stuff my smoothies full of 200 different ingredients. My digestion, while not perfect, is so much better. I'm able to eat without pain almost daily except for when I'm in a flare-up, and my acid reflux is basically gone. You taught me to question things and that what's on social media isn't always what's healthiest for every person! Thank you!

—Ava, 19

them completely for an extended period of time, you're more likely to have that "Aha!" moment when you try them later. (And if the food doesn't turn out to be an irritant for you, well, that's valuable info, too!)

Convinced yet? I hope so!

THE RIGHT COOKING TOOLS

Yes, I said cooking. Because part of the Gut Reset is preparing food for yourself. And if that's something you rarely (or never!) do, that's something I want you to start doing.

First, cooking for yourself is a powerful way to say "I matter." I started cooking for myself because I wanted to stop eating crap, basically. But I didn't realize how therapeutic it would be for me, and the positive impact it would have on how I felt. Like I said, I might not be able to control having IBS, but I could (and can) control what I choose to prepare, and cook, and eat—and that was a huge step in the right direction.

And cooking for myself was not only therapeutic; it also made me realize how many unnecessary ingredients companies add to their own products. I learned that I could make bread with simple, everyday ingredients I had in my pantry—the idea of having ten (or more!) ingredients in a "healthy" bread was just unnecessary. Plus, I ended up saving money, and my taste buds began to change and "normalize." I started to appreciate and actually *taste* the real food in the meal I created. Yes, of

course it was helping heal my gut and keep inflammation at bay, but it completely changed my way of thinking, tasting, and enjoying food!

Another thing? When you learn how to cook, you're constantly learning about what you enjoy, what you like, and what you don't like. Trust me—I wasn't a good cook at first. But the more time I spent in the kitchen, experimenting with different foods and different combinations and different techniques, the more fun I started to have.

Plus, I love food! I love coming up with different combinations, or devising my own, gut-friendly versions of favorite recipes I thought I could never have again. And you will, too. (And if coming up with recipes isn't your thing, not to worry—I've got you covered in the following chapters!)

Okay, so what equipment do you need in your kitchen? Honestly, there aren't that many essentials, but here are a few items you really should have on hand:

- **A good-quality blender.** Personally, I recommend a Vitamix. They're pricey but well worth the expense. I've had mine since 2014, and I still use it at least three times a day, every day! If you invest in only one thing, a Vitamix would be it!

- **An air fryer.** These are super useful, for so many reasons. They cut cooking time in half. They require little to no oil for when you want to create a good "fried" food. And they're easy to clean, which makes it more desirable for you to cook!

65

- **A small "bullet" blender.** This is a great option for making dips, spreads, and small amounts of purees.

- **A potato peeler.** This kitchen basic is great for taking the skins off cucumbers and hard-to-digest fruits and veggies.

- **"Stasher" bags.** These are reusable bags (not plastic bags) that you use to freeze your produce for smoothies. They may seem costly at first (for a bag), but they end up paying for themselves in a short time—plus you're producing less plastic waste!

THE GUT RESET FOODS

Okay, your mindset is ready. You've got what you need to cook the meals you'll eat. What's next? The food you need to successfully complete the Gut Reset program! Remember that what you *don't* eat is as important as what you *do* eat, so you may want to get rid of any Gut Irritants if they are foods you have a hard time saying no to. That includes known Gut Irritants like highly processed junk food and crap. Come on—you know what's bad for you!

Remember that if you eat any gut-irritating foods during the three weeks, you'll undo much, if not all, the progress you've made and you will have to start over. So, plan for success by stocking your pantry and refrigerator with the following:

- Grass-fed organic beef, pasture-raised organic chicken, and/or pasture-raised organic turkey. (You'll eat ½ cup to 1 cup a day, but no more than ½ cup at a time.)

- Plain whole-milk cultured Greek yogurt. Look for "organic" and "grass-fed" on the label, and make sure it contains no thickeners, gums, or sweeteners.

- Fresh kiwifruit, papaya, pineapple, and mango for the Digestive Boost (page 101).

- Brown or white rice, to eat with the yogurt. (You'll eat about ½ cup a day.)

- Bone broth. (Don't confuse it with beef stock or chicken stock!) Look for "grass-fed" or "pasture-raised" and "no additives" on the label; it's often near the frozen section. (You'll consume 1 to 3 cups a day.)

- Collagen. Look for "grass-fed" on the label, and make sure it only contains collagen as the single ingredient—such as "grass-fed bovine collagen peptides." (You'll consume 2 to 4 tablespoons per day.)

- Gelatin. As with collagen, look for "grass-fed" on the label and that it contains just one ingredient, like "grass-fed bovine gelatin."

- L-glutamine. Check the label to ascertain no additives, fillers, gums, or sweeteners; it should only contain one ingredient. (You'll take 1 teaspoon twice a day.)

NUT AND SEED BUTTERS: NOT NECESSARY, BUT HELPFUL

While the rules of the Gut Reset are fairly strict, I give you some leeway on nut and seed butters. You'll find them in some of the smoothie recipes. Nut and seed butters contain healthy fats, which improve satiety and help your body absorb fat-soluble vitamins. They're Gut Neutrals, which makes them acceptable to eat during the Gut Reset—and afterward! Just be sure to choose nut and seed butters that contain only the nut or seed it is made from, and opt for the "smooth" ones (instead of chunky) to avoid irritating your gut. Once again, it pays to read the labels!

- Probiotic protein powder of choice. (I recommend Probiotic Cacao Nuzest Protein Powder, my branded protein, which contains digestive enzymes, as well as L-glutamine. It's great for adding to smoothies—and you can mix it with water for a quick snack or dessert.)

- Nut and seed butters, if desired.

Take a look at chapter 7, which contains smoothie recipes, and make sure that you have the ingredients on hand to make a variety of smoothies. I can't say enough about smoothies. They're great go-tos when you need quick, nutritious meals, and they're a way to jam-pack a ton of nutrients into a small amount of food.

In addition to the Gut Reset basics, here are some foods that you may want to have on hand at home:

- Avocados

- Blanched almond flour (almond flour made without the skins)

- Cauliflower

- Cucumbers

- Frozen fruit (like cherries, strawberries, wild blueberries)

- Nut and seed butters (like SunButter, almond, cashew, tahini)

- Oil for cooking (avocado or coconut)

- Sweet potatoes

- Unsweetened cocoa powder and unsweetened chocolate (be sure it contains no other ingredients)

- Winter squash (acorn, butternut, delicata, spaghetti)

- Zucchini

MY SHORT LIST: SPECIFIC PRODUCTS I LOVE, USE, AND RECOMMEND

I have spent years tasting, testing, and developing recipes, and during that time I admit that I've developed some "faves." Here are some of the specific products I recommend:

- **Digestive Support Probiotic Nuzest Protein Powder and other Nuzest protein powders,** sold at www.nuzest-usa.com and select specialty health food stores

- **Vital Proteins unflavored collagen, gelatin, and bone broth powders,** sold at www.vitalproteins.com, select specialty health food stores, and major retailers like Amazon.com, Target, Walmart, Whole Foods, and Sprouts

- **Evo Hemp CBD, hemp protein powder, fruit and nut bars, and hemp seeds,** sold at www.evo-hemp.com

- **Organic SunButter,** sold at Amazon.com, Whole Foods, Sprouts, and select specialty health food stores

SMOOTHIES: YOUR GUT'S SECRET WEAPON

So, what else can you eat during the Gut Reset? Smoothies, smoothies, and more smoothies! I think you may have figured out that I love smoothies, but why? (Besides the fact that they taste like ice cream.) Smoothies are foods that are already broken down, so your gut has to do less work to digest them. Your gut has already been taxed, and the last thing you want to do is give it more work. Smoothies are not only easy to digest; they can even help soothe the stomach. If you've ever had ice cream after a spicy meal, you know what I mean. In a way, smoothies help calm the gut, all while giving your body the nutrients it needs to repair, replenish, and thrive!

SMOOTHIE PREP 101

Want to make it even easier to have nutritious, delicious smoothies? Do your smoothie prep ahead of time. Here's a list of some of my favorite smoothie ingredients, how to prepare them, and why I include them in the Gut Reset.

YOGURT

HOW TO PREPARE IT: Buy it, choosing plain, full-fat, whole-milk Greek yogurt with no additives.

WHY I LIKE IT: Yogurt provides smoothies with a creaminess without watering them down.

BENEFITS: As you know, it's a gut healer. It also adds protein, calcium, and probiotics to your smoothie, and the fat content helps you feel full longer.

PAPAYA

HOW TO PREPARE IT: Wash the outside first; even though you may not eat the outside of produce, it contains bacteria, and when you slice into the edible part, it can get contaminated. Slice it, remove the seeds (they're edible but are spicy-tasting), peel the skin, chop the flesh into cubes, and freeze.

WHY I LIKE IT: It adds a creaminess like no other!

BENEFITS: Papaya contains the digestive enzyme papain, which is specifically targeted to help digest protein.

BEETS

HOW TO PREPARE THEM: Wash them well and trim the root and stem ends. Steam them until you can pierce a fork into the centers; chop into cubes and freeze.

WHY I LIKE THEM: Beets add a natural sweetness to smoothies and they taste amazing (at least I think so!).

BENEFITS: Beets are a naturally detoxing root that helps cleanse the body. Just limit beets to ¼ cup or less at a time to avoid any digestive upset.

CUCUMBERS

HOW TO PREPARE THEM: Wash the outside of the cucumbers and take off the skin with a potato peeler. Discard the skins, as they can be very irritating to the gut. Chop the rest into cubes and freeze.

WHY I LIKE THEM: Cucumbers add volume to smoothies, thickening them without watering them down the way ice does.

BENEFITS: Cucumbers are super high in water content, so adding them to smoothies helps keep you hydrated and sneak in some extra H_2O! They also have a soothing effect on the stomach.

CAULIFLOWER

HOW TO PREPARE IT: Wash it, chop it, steam it until tender, and allow it to cool before freezing. (You can also put the steamed cauliflower in the freezer on a sheet tray for 30 minutes to cool down before placing it in a container or bag of choice to store in the freezer. If you do this, store pre-steamed/cooled cauliflower in a baggie, leaving "wiggle room" so it doesn't stick together in one large solid clump.)

WHY I LIKE IT: Cauliflower gives you tons of volume and creaminess without watering down your smoothie. (Not a cauliflower fan? Guess what—you won't even taste it in your smoothie.)

BENEFITS: Cauliflower is filled with nutrients, fiber, antioxidants, and choline, an essential nutrient. It can cause gas, but steaming it helps reduce the amount of gas it produces.

APPLES

HOW TO PREPARE THEM: I leave the skins on apples when I blend them, but you can peel the skins if you prefer. Wash the apples well, chop them, and freeze them.

WHY I LIKE THEM: Apples obviously taste amazing (my favorites are Pink Lady and Red Rome). And they contain the fiber called pectin.

BENEFITS: The pectin found in fruits, especially apples, has been used to treat conditions including constipation, diarrhea, high cholesterol, IBS (yup!), and ulcerative colitis.

DELICATA SQUASH

HOW TO PREPARE IT: Wash the outside well, slice horizontally, place on a roasting sheet face down, and roast at 350°F for about 40 minutes, or until the squash is fork-tender. Allow it to cool completely, then run a fork down the middle to remove seeds. Chop the flesh into cubes and freeze,

FROZEN VERSUS FRESH: DOES IT MATTER?

The suggestions starting on page 69 are some of my favorite gut-building smoothie ingredients, but that's just a selection of what is out there! Fruits and veggies are loaded with nutrients like the phytochemicals that your body craves—so much better for you than packaged "health food."

I like to buy as much fresh produce in season as possible, so when they are available, I chop and freeze peaches, cranberries, cherries (yes, I pit each one by hand), plums, butternut squash, zucchini, pumpkin, sweet potatoes, green bananas, and persimmons—you name it. (Green bananas have more resistant starch than ripe ones, which means they're absorbed more slowly by your body. That resistant starch also helps feed the probiotic bacteria in your gut. So, it's win-win when it comes to green bananas over ripe, at least for me.)

However, I also buy some frozen fruits so I have them on hand even when they're not in season. On any given day, you'll find frozen wild blueberries, cherries (if they're not in season), and cranberries (when I can't find them fresh) in my freezer. If you buy frozen fruits or veggies, just make sure they contain the fruit alone, with no added sugar or other ingredients.

using a big enough bag or container to prevent it from clumping into one giant mass.

WHY I LIKE IT: It tastes amazing! Delicata squash is also one of the rare winter squashes with edible skin (and that means less time prepping! Ha ha!). The skins are very thin, and I've had no trouble digesting them.

BENEFITS: Delicata squash contains a good amount of vitamin C, calcium, and iron.

BUTTERNUT SQUASH

HOW TO PREPARE IT: Wash the outside well, cut off the ends, and then slice horizontally and place on a roasting sheet facedown and roast at 350°F for about 40 minutes, or until the squash is fork-tender. Allow it to cool completely, then carefully remove the seeds. Chop the flesh into cubes and freeze, using a big enough bag or container to prevent them from clumping into one giant mass.

WHY I LIKE IT: Butternut squash is available year-round, so having it on hand is never an issue. It's also slightly sweet yet still low in sugar. Plus, you can save the round end pieces and stuff them with quinoa, rice, or yogurt with a light drizzle of raw honey! So good!

BENEFITS: Butternut squash is high in potassium, vitamin C, and vitamin A (great for eye health!).

SWEET POTATOES

HOW TO PREPARE THEM: Wash the outside well and use a potato peeler to remove the skins (you can leave the skins on but if your tummy is sensitive right now, it's best to remove them) and chop into 1-inch cubes. Place cubes in a steamer or boil them in water for about 15 minutes, or until they are fork-tender. Allow to cool completely. For freezing, place cooled sweet potato cubes in a big enough bag or container to prevent them from forming a giant mass.

WHY I LIKE THEM: Sweet potatoes are sweet! (no duh!). But they can actually be used in many savory applications too, like main dishes, snacks, and desserts! The possibilities are endless!

BENEFITS: Sweet potatoes are packed with antioxidants and contain natural anti-inflammatory compounds. And because of their slow-burning starches, they won't spike your blood sugar levels.

STRAWBERRIES

HOW TO PREPARE THEM: Wash them well, remove the hulls, chop the berries, and freeze.

WHY I LIKE THEM: Despite what you might think, strawberries are actually very low in sugar. One entire cup contains just 7 grams of natural sugar, but to me they taste extra sweet! Win-win!

BENEFITS: Eight average strawberries contain more vitamin C than an orange! If the seeds on the outside bother you (for example, if you have diverticulitis), either avoid strawberries completely or blend them extremely well to break up the seeds before adding them to your smoothie. (If you have a Vitamix, this shouldn't be an issue.)

71

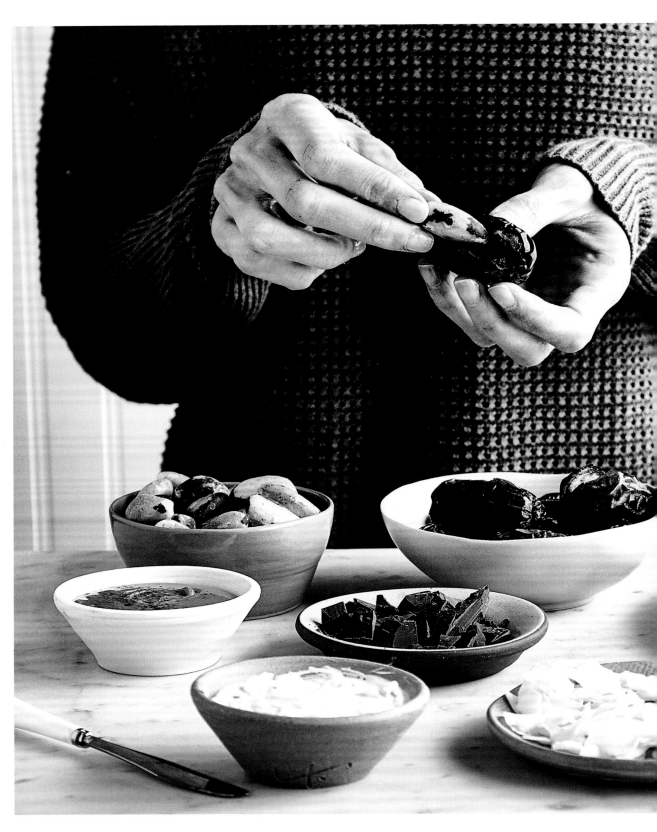

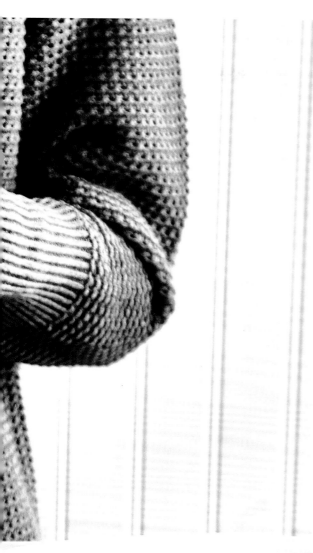

BEFORE YOU BEGIN: CHECKING IN

There's one more thing I want you to do before you begin the Gut Reset, and that's to get clear about how you're feeling day to day, right now. I've found that it's too easy to forget how you felt at any given point in time, or that you may exaggerate how bad your symptoms were—or even downplay how much they affected your life!

Use the checklist on page 74 to make a note of how you feel now. If you like, you can make copies of the page and track how you feel over several days.

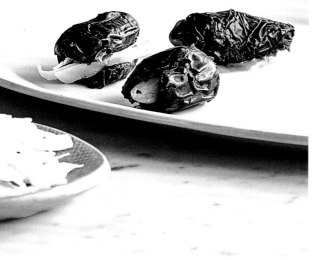

PRE-GUT RESET

BREAKFAST:

How well do you sleep? How do you feel when you wake up? And how do you feel before breakfast? Are you in pain from the night before? Or is this your "best-feeling" time of the day? _____

_____

_____

What is your typical breakfast? _____

_____

_____

What's your typical morning like? Are you in a rush? Are you preoccupied with work or what you need to get done? _____

_____

_____

How do you typically feel after break-fast? (Bloated, gassy, headachy, energized, satisfied, fatigued, etc.) _____

_____

_____

_____

_____

_____

_____

MID-MORNING SNACK:

Are you usually hungry at this time? How do you feel physically and emotionally?

_____

_____

Do have you a snack mid-morning? If so, what is it and how do you feel afterward?

_____

_____

LUNCH:

What do you typically have for lunch? _____

_____

_____

_____

Do you usually eat lunch in a rush, or while working? _____

_____

_____

Do you usually eat lunch with other people, or alone? _____

_____

_____

How do feel after this meal? _____

_____

_____

AFTERNOON SNACK:

Do you typically have an afternoon snack? If so, what is it?

Do you often eat snacks while in a rush, in the car, and "on the go"?

How do you feel after this snack?

DINNER:

What do you typically eat for dinner?

Do you usually eat alone or with others?

What do you do while you're eating? Are you in a rush, for example?

How do you feel after this meal?

NOTES OF THE DAY:

How are your bathroom habits in a typical day?

Are there certain situations or emotions that seem to trigger digestive upset, bloating, cramping, diarrhea, etc.? What are they?

In a typical day, does anything tend to trigger anger, frustration, stress, or other negative emotions?
If so, what time of the day does this typically happen? Is it around the time of any of your meals or snacks?

In a typical day, do you take time to do something positive for yourself? If so, what kinds of things do you do?

75

DURING THE GUT RESET

Answer these questions during each of the 21 days of the Gut Reset.

BREAKFAST:

How well did you sleep? How did you feel when you woke up? Are you in pain from the night before? Or was this your "best-feeling" time of the day? _____

_____

What did you have for breakfast? _____

_____

_____

Did you remember to turn on the parasympathetic nervous system before you ate?

_____

_____

How did you feel before breakfast? How did you feel afterward? (Bloated, gassy, headachy, energized, satisfied, fatigued, etc.) ____

_____

_____

_____

_____

_____

_____

MID-MORNING SNACK:

Are you usually hungry at this time? How do you feel physically and emotionally?

_____

_____

Did you remember to turn on the parasympathetic nervous system before you ate?

_____

_____

What did you have for a snack? How did you feel afterward? _____

_____

_____

LUNCH:

What did you have for lunch? _____

_____

_____

Did you remember to turn on the parasympathetic nervous system before you ate?

_____

_____

How did you feel before lunch? How did you feel afterward? (Bloated, gassy, headachy, energized, satisfied, fatigued, etc.) _____

_____

_____

_____

AFTERNOON SNACK:

What did you have for a snack?

Did you remember to turn on the parasympathetic nervous system before you ate?

How did you feel before your snack? How did you feel afterward? (Bloated, gassy, headachy, energized, satisfied, fatigued, etc.)

DINNER:

What did you have for dinner?

Did you remember to turn on the parasympathetic nervous system before you ate?

How did you feel before dinner? How did you feel afterward? (Bloated, gassy, headachy, energized, satisfied, fatigued, etc.)

NOTES OF THE DAY:

How were your bathroom habits today?

Did you have any digestive symptoms throughout the day? If so, what were they?

Did anything happen today that caused anger, frustration, stress, or other negative emotions? What happened?

Did this in turn trigger digestive upset, bloating, cramping, diarrhea, etc?

Did it happen around the time you ate meals or snacks?

Note anything you did or did not like about any of the meals and snacks above. In three weeks, you should look back on your notes from the earliest days. Your taste buds most likely will have changed!

Did you perform some type of stress management technique today, or otherwise do something positive for yourself? What did you do?

How did you feel afterward?

Did anything positive happen that gave you joy today?

If so, think about that and be thankful for it! Dwell on it!

Additional thoughts about today—about how you felt physically and emotionally (take as much space as you need to write about any changes, both positive and negative, you're experiencing):

A TYPICAL DAY ON THE GUT RESET

So, you've got the basics down. You've got the food you need. You know how you felt on a typical day, and you're ready to heal and seal your gut. Maybe you're a little nervous. Don't worry—I've got you covered! Remember, you want to have some pureed protein, plain whole-milk yogurt, Digestive Boost (page 101), and either gelatin or collagen every day. (Remember, you'll get the latter in smoothies and other recipes.) And don't forget to take a few moments to settle into a parasympathetic state before you start eating. Here's what one week on the Gut Reset might look like.

MONDAY

Breakfast: ½ cup of Digestive Boost (page 101), ¼ cup of pureed chicken

Mid-morning snack: Protein Fluff (page 195), 2 tablespoons of unsweetened chocolate chips

Lunch: Smoothie of choice

Afternoon snack: ¼ cup of pureed chicken

Dinner: Smoothie of choice or Sweet Pea Gazpacho (page 131)

TUESDAY

Breakfast: Creamy Morning Matcha (page 212); ½ cup of the Digestive Boost (page 101)

Mid-morning snack: Protein Fluff (page 195), 1 tablespoon of creamy almond or cashew butter

Lunch: Smoothie of choice

Afternoon snack: ¼ cup of pureed chicken

Dinner: Smoothie of choice

WEDNESDAY

Breakfast: ½ cup of Digestive Boost (page 101), ¼ cup of pureed chicken

Mid-morning snack: ½ cup of Digestive Boost (page 101)

Lunch: Smoothie of choice

Afternoon snack: Protein Fluff (page 195)

Dinner: Sweat Pea Gazpacho (page 131) or smoothie of choice

THURSDAY

Breakfast: Gut-Healing Frothy Coffee (page 216); ¼ cup pureed chicken

Mid-morning snack: ½ cup of Digestive Boost (page 101)

Lunch: Smoothie of choice

Afternoon snack: Protein Fluff (page 195), 2 tablespoons of unsweetened chocolate chips

Dinner: Sweet Pea Gazpacho (page 131)

FRIDAY

Breakfast: Gut-Healing Frothy Coffee (page 216); ¼ cup of pureed chicken

Mid-morning snack: ½ cup of Digestive Boost (page 101)

Lunch: Smoothie of choice

Afternoon snack: Protein Fluff (page 195) and 1 tablespoon of creamy nut or seed butter

Dinner: Smoothie of choice

SATURDAY

Breakfast: Gut-Healing Frothy Coffee (page 216); ¼ cup of pureed chicken

Mid-morning snack: ½ cup of Digestive Boost (page 101)

Lunch: Smoothie of choice

Afternoon snack: Protein Fluff (page 195) and 1 tablespoon of creamy almond butter

Dinner: Smoothie of choice or Butternut Squash and Apple Soup (page 160)

SUNDAY

Breakfast: ½ cup of the Digestive Boost (page 101), ¼ cup of pureed chicken

Mid-morning snack: Protein Fluff (page 195), 2 tablespoons of unsweetened chocolate chips

Lunch: Smoothie of choice

Afternoon snack: ¼ cup of unsweetened applesauce with 1 tablespoon of creamy SunButter

Dinner: Smoothie of choice or Butternut Squash and Apple Soup (page 160)

MOVING ON...

What's my last word on the Gut Reset? *Consistency*. Keep at it and stick with it. Remember, this is just for a short period of time and you don't have to live this way forever.

I promise that a few days into the program, you'll find that your new eating habits will have become routine. What may not be routine is the freedom from symptoms you may have had for years. Track what you eat, and how you feel, during this 21-day period so that you can trace your improvement. In the next chapter, I suggest you do the same thing, as you add back some foods into your diet to see how they make you feel. Remember: When you finish the Gut Reset, the hardest part of the *Digest This* plan is behind you. Next up is the rest of your life!

SHOPPING LIST

PRODUCE

1 large Mexican papaya

1 medium pineapple

1 large mango

3 medium kiwifruits

4 large Honeycrisp apples

1 avocado

1 large butternut squash

3 medium sweet potatoes

1 head of cauliflower

6 large cucumbers

6 large zucchini

1 16-ounce bag of frozen cherries

1 16-ounce bag of frozen peas

MEAT/FISH

3 organic chicken breasts

DAIRY

3 35-ounce tubs of plain whole-milk Greek yogurt, such as Fage

CANNED/ JARRED GOODS

1 8-ounce jar of grass-fed ghee (clarified butter)

1 8-ounce jar of coconut oil

1 16-ounce jar of organic SunButter

1 16-ounce jar of cashew butter

1 16-ounce jar of creamy almond butter

1 4-ounce 4-pack of unsweetened applesauce

1 8-ounce jar of raw honey

1 15-ounce bottle unsulfured blackstrap molasses

DRIED GOODS/ PANTRY ITEMS

1 12-ounce bag of organic coffee

1 17-ounce tub of protein powder (such as my Digestive Support Probiotic Nuzest Protein Powder)

1 32-ounce tub of grass-fed gelatin, such as Vital Proteins

1 20-ounce tub of grass-fed collagen peptides, such as Vital Proteins

8 ounces of unsweetened chocolate chips

1 pound of unsweetened cacao powder

AFTER THE GUT RESET:
ENJOYING YOUR HEALTHY GUT—FOR LIFE

Congratulations! You've made it! Those three weeks may have been rough, but you did it. You've cleared your gut of irritants that were no doubt causing issues, and you are now on the path to continued healing and to sealing your gut, restoring your microbiome, and building on this foundation for a healthy digestive system.

Now that you've reset your gut, you can have more freedom with your diet. This is the maintenance phase of the program—the time to add foods to your diet, paying attention to how you react to them. You may find that now that your gut is healthy, foods that formerly bothered you are no longer an issue. However, there may be some foods that still cause bloating, discomfort, and other digestive issues. We all get bloated from time to time, but there is a difference between the occasional bloating and the kind of bloating that causes you to bend over with so much pain you can't even think. That is something we are working to rid ourselves of once and for all!

You'll learn to introduce these new foods in a bit. But first, I want to review the behavioral principles #7 and #8–of the *Digest This* plan. To refresh your memory, those are:

- **Principle #7:** Turn on the parasympathetic nervous system before you eat. This helps trigger the "rest and digest" parasympathetic system, which helps lower stress hormones like cortisol and adrenaline, and improves digestive function.

- **Principle #8:** Perform at least one stress-reduction technique every day.

Because the brain–gut connection plays a factor in IBS, managing the stress you feel on a daily basis can have a powerful impact on your overall digestive health.

MAKING FRIENDS WITH YOUR PARA-SYMPATHETIC SYSTEM

You know now that gut problems aren't just related to what you eat and how you eat. Your dominant nervous system will dictate how well your body digests the food and absorbs the nutrients. If your sympathetic nervous system is switched on–as it is when you're stressed, anxious, or upset–you won't be able to digest food the way you need to. When your parasympathetic nervous system is switched on, however, you'll lower the level of stress hormones, slow your heart rate and lower your blood pressure, and improve your digestion.

Let's recap what you learned last chapter. When your sympathetic nervous system is activated, your body responds by sending blood away from your digestive system and to your limbs—in case you need to fight off an attacker, or run away. Your heart rate, breathing, and blood pressure all increase. You produce less saliva, and your body hits "pause" on digesting food. If you're eating when the sympathetic system is activated, you're asking your body to do the opposite of what it's primed to do.

Now, when your parasympathetic system is activated, your body prepares itself to rest and digest. Your breathing and heart rate slow. Your muscles relax. You produce more saliva, digestive enzymes are released, and your body prepares to digest any available food. When the parasympathetic system is activated, your body is relaxed and unstressed.

Now, ask yourself: How often do you feel that kind of "unstressed" feeling? Do you feel it ever? I know that today's go-go-go world means that you may always feel like you're trying to get something done; and when you're "relaxing," you're probably staring at a screen. (Here's a tip: All that time on your phone, even on social media, isn't good for your brain in terms of stress or in turning on your parasympathetic system. Well, if you're listening to a meditation app, I'll give you a pass. But anyway…)

So, what I want you to do is to learn how to turn on your parasympathetic system as often as you can—not only before you eat but also at different times during the day. I also want you to embrace principle #8 of practicing stress-reduction techniques regularly—at least once a day. First, these kinds of de-stressing strategies work and can turn on your parasympathetic system. But they have another advantage, too: by doing them regularly, you increase your body's resistance to stress. In other words, it makes it harder for you to turn on your "fight or flight" sympathetic nervous system. And that is good!

You may already know this intuitively. Think about how you feel after a session of yoga or a fun night out with a friend, during which you talked and laughed for hours, or how you felt after meditating. (Don't know how? Don't worry—I'm going to show you.) You feel relaxed. Content. Like nothing can bother you and get you down.

Well, that's how you feel when your parasympathetic system is activated, and the more you activate it, the easier it becomes to access it—even in the middle of a busy, stressed-out day! And just as stress is linked to IBS symptoms, lowering your stress levels is associated with fewer symptoms of IBS—and improvement in overall symptom severity.

Remember that while your sympathetic nervous system has an important role, the more often it is activated, the less healthy you're likely to be—not only in terms of your gut health but of your overall health as well. Chronic stress, or your body's perception of stress, is linked with about 75 percent of all health problems—everything from heart disease, to high blood pressure, to immune suppression, to digestive problems, cold sores, and anxiety. It's that prevalent, and that dangerous.

Yes, you want to feel some anxiety before an important presentation at work or to feel motivated to find a job when you don't have one. A little bit of stress is good! A lot of stress, or even a little bit of stress all of the time, is not good. The bottom line? The more time you spend with the parasympathetic system in charge, the better. So, just how do you do that?

STRESS-MANAGEMENT TECHNIQUES

When it comes to stress management, what works for you may not work for someone else, and vice versa. That means you really have to know, or figure out, what will work for you. I've found the following techniques to be useful, and they should help you as well!

CHANGE YOUR MINDSET

When I talk about stress, you probably think of the outside things that make you nuts—your job, your family, too many responsibil-ities, not enough money, conflicting obligations, you name it. But a primary source of stress—maybe the primary cause of stress—comes from inside you. It's your mindset.

Think about it. Stress isn't what happens to you—it's how you react to what happens.

Let's say you're running 15 minutes late to meet a friend for dinner. This makes some people stressed and upset. But for other people, the same situation might not cause any distress. "I'll get there when I get there," one might think, and the person doesn't even stress over it. See what I mean? It's not what happens that is stressful. It's how you interpret and react to the event that determines whether you'll find it stressful. I admit I used to stress about a lot of things!

One thing I think we can all relate to is stressing over food. If I'm going to a party or gathering, I sometimes get stressed out about whether there is going to be food there for me to eat that won't upset my gut. Or often, when I get an IBS flare-up, I stress over the situation (which makes it worse!) and then it becomes a never-ending cycle: stress > IBS flare-up > stressing about the flare-up > stress gets worse.

So, how do you change your mindset? *By accepting things you cannot change.* IBS is a good example of this! You can't help whether you have IBS or other digestive problems. Worrying about it or being angry about it won't help—and in fact may make your symptoms worse.

There's a lot in your life you can't change! Let's say you are running late for dinner—and there isn't anything you can do about it. You can let yourself feel angry and irritated, or you can decide to go with the flow and move on. If there's traffic, learn to enjoy what you can and make the best of it. Think, *Hmmm, now's a perfect time to listen to that podcast I've been wanting to hear.*

One thing I've learned being so active on social media is that we have no control over how other people act or think, or whether they like or respect or agree with us. You know what I do? I focus on doing what I love to do—creating out-of-the-box recipes and sharing them and my personal story with the world, and connecting with my followers, friends, and family—and let go of worrying about everything else.

Of course, sometimes that's a lot easier to do than at other times. So, changing your mindset is one part of managing stress, but sometimes you will feel overwhelmed, anxious, angry, or depressed. That's life! When you feel overwhelmed, it can help to remind yourself that all emotions—even the strongest or scariest—are only temporary. They do pass.

MEDITATION

Changing your mindset can help you be less reactive to stress, but one of the easiest—and most effective—ways to manage stress is meditation. No, you don't have to sit cross-legged or chant a mantra. Start by sitting in a comfortable position, and pay attention to your breath. Inhale slowly and comfortably and exhale slowly as well. If you like, place your hand on your belly; your belly should swell a little as you inhale and retract a bit as you exhale. Close your eyes and focus on your breath for a few minutes.

When thoughts come into your mind, try to simply notice them without engaging them. Pretend like they are simply clouds passing by in the sky and that you can notice them without stopping to question or explore them. You should feel your heart rate slow down as your breathing slows down. Start by meditating for five minutes at first, working up to longer stretches of time as you get more comfortable "sitting."

And don't give up if the first couple of times it's hard to sit quietly, without thinking about all of the things you could be doing! It's normal to feel a little overwhelmed or uncomfortable at first—most of us are used to being constantly on the go, run-run-running all day and rarely taking the time to simply sit. But research shows that regular meditation helps us manage stress more effectively, because it helps reduce the body's overall stress response.

Still not convinced? If you pray, take a few minutes for prayer. Or take a walk and make a mental gratitude list, recognizing all the good things you have in your life. The more often you use techniques like these, the better able you will be to withstand all the pressures of your day-to-day life, including the

CAN CHIROPRACTIC HELP DIGESTION?

It never occurred to me that being in proper alignment could actually affect digestion (negatively and positively). But once I started chiropractic care and experienced the benefits, I was sold and, of course, had to dig deeper as to *why*. Think about it: The digestive system is linked to the nervous system (as with everything), and the brain sends signals to the nerves through the spinal cord to determine when to eliminate stool. If your body is out of alignment, these nerves can be pinched and compressed, interfering with the signal flow.

Regular chiropractic care may help alleviate digestive discomfort by adjusting the bones and muscles that are directly connected to the stomach and other digestive organs. It can even help with headaches! There have been times when I was eating all the right foods, doing all the right things, but still was experiencing an IBS flare-up. I came to find out my nerves were pinched from a workout I did a few days prior, and within an hour of getting adjusted I could certainly feel my digestive juices flowing again. It's crazy how our body parts are so connected!

stress of having IBS. And when you are less stressed and less reactive, you're likely to have fewer symptoms as well. A win-win!

BREAK THE STRESS HABIT

During the 21 days of the Gut Reset, you were supposed to stop and take a few minutes to turn on the parasympathetic nervous system before you ate. You did that for three weeks, five times a day, or 105 times! That is more than 100 times you taught your body how to relax, even for a few minutes. Great work!

You know what happens when you turn on the parasympathetic system more frequently? Just as with meditation, it gets easier to do. You find that you relax more quickly, and more deeply, than you could before. But sometimes you need more than a few minutes of deep breathing or relaxing reading to work out all that stress. That's why regular stress-management techniques are so important. Whether or not you choose to meditate (though I hope you'll at least try it), I want you to do at least one activity that you enjoy and is good for you, every day.

Whether you exercise, pray, read, journal, listen to music, connect with friends, cook, or even clean—it doesn't matter what you do. All that matters is that you enjoy it and that it gives you a break from the day-to-day pressure we all face. When you do it regularly, something amazing happens. You become more resistant to stress, or more properly, you become more resistant to the types of things that used to cause you stress.

And as you become more resistant to stress, your digestive system does, too. That means that an important meeting or hot date (ha ha!) is less likely to cause gas or bloating or unexpected runs to the bathroom. And that is the goal of the whole *Digest This* plan, after all: to heal your gut. You already know that your gut and your brain are closely linked. Use that as a motivator when you consider skipping that yoga class or shorting yourself on sleep. Look at your stress management as an essential part of your overall health and wellness. It's that important, especially when you're dealing with IBS.

SLEEP AND IBS: MAKING IT A PRIORITY

There's another aspect of stress management that's important to consider: your sleep. If you have IBS, there is a good chance that you have sleep issues, too. Here's the thing: When you have IBS, it is also likely to affect the quality of your sleep. (If you have anxiety or depression, you're also more likely to have sleep problems.) People with IBS are about 1.6 times more likely to have trouble falling asleep, more likely to have trouble staying asleep, more likely to wake up frequently at night, and more likely to not feel rested in the morning than people without IBS. If you have IBS, you are also more likely to have to get up in the middle of the night to use the bathroom for a bowel movement. I used to have horrible stomach pains that would keep me up all night, not allowing my body to rest, and in turn, that would disrupt my digestion (and life) the next day—it was a vicious cycle.

Researchers are looking into the connection between sleep disturbances and IBS. If you have a bad night of sleep, you're more likely to have bad IBS symptoms the next day. However, having symptoms during the day doesn't necessarily mean that you'll sleep poorly that night. So, there is some good news!

What can you do in the meantime? Make sleep a priority by trying the following:

- **Set the stage.** Studies show that you sleep best in a cool, dark, quiet room.

- **Stick to a regular routine.** Sure, it's tempting to sleep in on weekends, especially if you get up early during the week, but it's better for your sleep habits to go to bed and get up at the same time every day.

- **Use sound to help you relax.** Try listening to instrumental music or rain sounds. You can find plenty of free playlists on YouTube designed for sleep. I personally love the sound of the ocean!

- **Try taking CBD 30 minutes before bed.** This has helped me tremendously. I have used Evo Hemp for the past three years and love that it's pure with no flavorings or sweeteners (which many brands now incorporate into their CBD tinctures, so be aware).

- **Don't go to bed hungry!** I actually have a little something like Greek yogurt, bone broth, or my probiotic Protein Fluff (page 195) an hour before bed. Doing something like this will help prevent you from waking up because you're hungry, and a high-protein snack will also help with muscle repair. Remember, your body is working 24/7 and burning calories while you sleep. Your organs need energy to do their work!

- **Avoid caffeine and alcohol.** First, both can mess with your sleep—and affect your gut function, too! Avoid them completely, or if you enjoy coffee or tea, have your last cup early in the afternoon to give your body a chance to clear the caffeine before bed. Alcohol may make you feel sleepy because it's a depressant, but when it wears off, it can affect your sleep quality.

- **Avoid naps!** If you're tired, it can be tempting to take a short snooze. A nap of 20 minutes or so may not affect your sleep that night, but sleeping longer than that can make it harder to fall and stay asleep.

- **Limit screen time.** The blue light from smartphones, tablets, computers, and even the good old TV can trick your brain into thinking it's still daylight and make it harder to fall asleep. Try investing in a pair of blue-light-blocking glasses; I have a couple pairs and certainly notice a difference when I wear them—not only in the quality of sleep but also in less strain on my eyes.

THE REST OF YOUR LIFE: ADDING MORE FOODS INTO YOUR REGULAR DIET

Okay. Now that you've finished the Gut Reset and have healed your gut, it's time to take the wheels off—but slowly. First, ask yourself how you feel. Are you tired of eating the same thing (even with all of those smoothies?) and ready to branch out into other foods? Or are you relieved to be free from most (if not all!) of the digestive symptoms you've been dealing with for years? Or maybe a little bit of both?

There are no right answers or right feelings here. I just want you to recognize and remember that food is emotionally loaded for people with perfectly normal, functioning digestive symptoms. For those of us with IBS, what we eat presents even more of an emotional minefield! But remember, the only way to learn about your gut, and what works for it and may not, is to experiment now with introducing foods, paying attention to what you eat and how you react to them.

Baby-step your way here! Ease your gut into new foods. For example, you might start with eating half a cooked chicken breast instead of having it pureed, gradually moving away from the pureed protein you've been consuming. (Note that you can continue to eat all the foods on the Gut Reset—it's just not required at this point.)

Ready to add foods to your routine? I recommend adding or trying a new food one at a time. For example, instead of having a smoothie for a meal, the way you did on the Gut Reset, try having a smaller smoothie as a snack and then progress to full-on "non-smoothie" meals. If you introduce too many foods at once, you can upset your gut; also, if something does cause an upset, you may not be able to determine what caused the reaction.

Keep in mind, though, that this isn't an excuse to go back to eating processed or crappy food loaded with additives (or known Gut Irritants)! The more you can base your diet on Gut Neutrals and Gut Healers, the better. One other thing to consider is that the longer you've been sick with IBS, the longer it likely will take to completely heal your gut—and the more reactive your gut may still be to irritating foods.

I suggest you continue using the food checklist pages in chapter 4 to track what you ate, when, and how you felt afterward, including any reactions you had. Also, feel free to start trying the recipes in the rest of this book, which have been developed for people with IBS, and do "tweak" them any way you like. Lastly, while I'm a big fan of eating fruits and veggies, there are some vegetables you should consume cooked (see page 91).

I do suggest that you keep smoothies as part of your regular diet. Smoothies give your gut a break. When food is pureed, your digestive system doesn't have to work as hard to break down the food, allowing your body to "save" energy. (Yes, it takes energy to break down food.) Not only that, but if you don't chew well, small particles may get stuck in your gut, which can cause inflammation, bloating, and gas, as the food is sitting and rotting inside your stomach. Yuck!

You don't have to eat smoothies every day now that your gut is better, but let me ask you this: Do you change your car's oil every day? No! Once it's had an oil change, your engine is good to go for a while and will run smoothly. It's the same with your gut. Smoothies are "upkeep" for your gut. If you don't maintain your gut health, "dirt" will accumulate in your system over time, just like a car engine's oil gets dirty over time.

If you change the oil in your car regularly (or, in this case, eat a smoothie every day), you keep your car (or your gut) functioning

VEGGIES TO EAT COOKED

There is nothing like the taste of fresh veggies, especially when you pick them up at a farmers' market. But while veggies like cucumbers, salad greens, and zucchini are all delicious raw, some vegetables should be cooked for better absorption in the body. Those veggies include:

- **Asparagus.** It won't harm you to consume asparagus raw, but cooking it helps your body absorb more of its cancer-fighting nutrients.
- **Mushrooms.** Mushrooms can be eaten raw, but you'll receive more of the veggie's benefits if you take the time to sauté, roast, or even grill them.
- **Tomatoes.** Obviously we eat raw tomatoes in salads, sandwiches, and salsa, but your body can absorb more of the cancer-fighting ingredient lycopene from cooked tomatoes. Try some grilled tomatoes in a sandwich!
- **Potatoes.** For some reason, I get asked a lot on social media, "Why can't I eat raw potatoes?" Um, well, they're toxic uncooked. That's why! Not only do raw potatoes contain toxins that can harm your body, but their uncooked starchiness can also cause digestive discomfort. (This applies to all non-sweet potatoes, including russet, waxy white, red, fingerling, and purple potatoes, which should not be confused with purple sweet potatoes.)
- **Brussels sprouts.** Brussels sprouts can cause gas and bloating if consumed raw. They're not toxic; however, they can cause a great deal of discomfort when eaten uncooked. For better digestion and absorption, steam, roast, or sauté with avocado oil.
- **Cauliflower.** I'm often asked why I steam my cauliflower before freezing for my smoothies. The fact is that steaming the cauliflower first helps you digest it better—and it produces less gas and bloating, as well. Try lightly steaming it to retain the liver-cleansing enzymes it contains!

optimally. You wouldn't put cheap oil in your car's engine because you know your engine won't function as well; so, too, choosing the right "oils" for your gut can improve its overall function. That's why I try to consume gelatin, collagen, and/or my Probiotic Cacao Nuzest Protein Powder every day.

These supplements are part of the Gut Reset, but I suggest you try taking them continually as part of your regular gut maintenance—every day if possible. I've been taking all three for literally years and will continue to. I prefer the Vital Proteins brand for the gelatin and collagen; the Nuzest brand is the only one I've collaborated with to create my own blend of digestive support. My goal here is to not only to help you have an optimum gut but also to give you the tools to make informed decisions so you can live an optimum life! Let me leave you with a thought, though. Your gut is now in the best shape it's been in months, maybe years. So, before you try a food that you know will cause you digestive upset, ask yourself whether it's worth the symptoms it may produce. Are you worried about people judging you, or making comments about what you're eating or not eating?

The people who truly care for you won't judge. They'll understand (or at least try to) what you need to do for yourself. People may not ever "get" or fully grasp your issues or experience what you've been through, but they will still accept you as a friend, partner, and family member. Indeed, most of the time these worries are in our own heads! We often overthink things and over-analyze how others view us. And if people have issues with how you eat (most likely they'll be jealous of all of the delicious foods you're making), the issue isn't with you. It's with them.

When I was feeling embarrassed about eating differently from others, I forgot to actually tell people why I was doing it. Once I started sharing my story and being more open about my circumstances, people understood and didn't think twice about why I was bringing my own food to gatherings or why I wasn't partaking in their meal. So, remember to tell people and share what you're going through. You may be surprised at the support and compassion you receive.

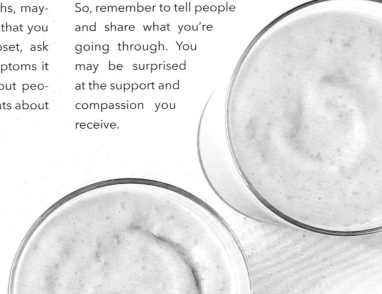

GET READY FOR THE RECIPES . . . AND MORE EAT-ING FREEDOM THAN EVER BEFORE!

One of the things that my followers love about my *Digest This* plan is that after the Gut Reset, there's no "official" program to follow. While I strongly encourage you to continue to take gelatin and collagen, and to enjoy a smoothie every day (or at least often!), really all you need to do is avoid the Gut Irritants you learned about in chapter 2; and to feed your gut the nutrient-dense, good-for-you foods that make up the recipes in this book. In other words, here comes the fun stuff!

Remember, I'm all about helping you find food freedom, so you're free to experiment and develop the eating plan that works for you after the Gut Reset. Obviously, if a certain food doesn't agree with you, you'll want to avoid it, but I encourage you to experiment. You may now find that foods that used to bother you can be consumed without any digestive issues. That's another sign that your gut is healing and sealing.

Here's what several days of eating per the *Digest This* guidelines might look like:

MONDAY

Breakfast: Gut-Healing Frothy Coffee (page 216), Soaked Chocolate Probiotic Oatmeal (page 135)

Snack: Easy-Peasy Protein Cookie Dough Bites (page 210)

Lunch: Lasagna Sandwich (page 166)

Snack: Protein Fluff (page 195), 1 tablespoon of nut or seed butter of choice

Dinner: Healthy Chinese "Takeout" (page 174)

Dessert: Sea Salt Butternut Fudge (page 241)

TUESDAY

Breakfast: Creamy Morning Matcha (page 212), Blueberry Protein Scones (page 136)

Snack: Protein Cake Batter Balls (page 202)

Lunch: Lasagna Sandwich (page 166)

Snack: Easy-Peasy Protein Cookie Dough Bites (page 210)

Dinner: Chilled Avocado–Cucumber Mint Soup (page 182)

Dessert: Protein Fluff (page 195), 2 tablespoons of chocolate chips, 1 tablespoon of SunButter

WEDNESDAY

Breakfast: Baked Breakfast Oatmeal Cookie (page 144), Coconut Coffee Cubes (page 142)

Snack: Low-Carb Chocolate Graham Crackers (page 198)

Lunch: Gut-Healing "PB&J" (page 153)

Snack: Blueberry Protein Scones (page 136)

Dinner: Better Than Mac 'n' Cheese (page 159)

Dessert: Carb-Free Crumb Cookies (page 226)

THURSDAY

Breakfast: Gut-Healing Frothy Coffee (page 216), Iced Pistachio Coconut Cake (page 141)

Snack: 1 Evo Hemp Fruit and Nut Bar

Lunch: Sweet Potato–Chocolate Cherry Smoothie (page 112)

Snack: Protein Fluff (page 195), 2 tablespoons chocolate chips, 1 tablespoon of SunButter

Dinner: Grilled (Cauliflower) "Cheese" Sandwich (page 163)

Dessert: Low-Carb Butternut Brownies (page 242)

FRIDAY

Breakfast: Creamy Morning Matcha (page 212), Iced Pistachio Coconut Cake (page 141)

Snack: Protein Cake Batter Balls (page 202)

Lunch: Baked Sweet Potato Fries with Sweet Yogurt Dipping Sauce (page 156)

Snack: Sea Salt Butternut Fudge (page 241)

Dinner: Butternut Squash and Apple Soup (page 160)

Dessert: Carb-Free Crumb Cookies (page 226)

SATURDAY

Breakfast: Gut-Healing Frothy Coffee (page 216), "Banilla" Bean Protein Pancake (page 147)

Snack: Low-Carb Chocolate Graham Crackers (page 198)

Lunch: Butternut Squash and Apple Soup (page 160)

Snack: 1 Evo Hemp Fruit and Nut Bar

Dinner: No-Cook Hemp Pasta Salad (page 158)

Dessert: Sea Salt Butternut Fudge (page 241)

SUNDAY

Breakfast: Gut-Healing Frothy Coffee (page 216), Five-Minute Egg Hemp Hash (page 151)

Snack: Protein Fluff (page 195), 2 tablespoons of chocolate chips, 1 tablespoon of SunButter

Lunch: No-Cook Hemp Pasta Salad (page 158)

Snack: Stuffed Dates (page 209)

Dinner: Stuffed Sweet Potato Taco (page 154)

Dessert: Low-Carb Butternut Brownies (page 242)

SHOPPING LIST

PRODUCE

1 16-ounce bag of frozen blueberries

1 16-ounce bag of frozen cherries

1 16-ounce bag of frozen mixed veggies

1 large Mexican papaya

4 large Honeycrisp apples

2 heads of cauliflower

1 8-ounce bag of frozen cauliflower rice

2 long carrots

5 large zucchini

5 large cucumbers

4 ounces of Medjool dates

1 sprig of fresh mint

1 sprig of fresh cilantro

2 large butternut squash

5 large sweet potatoes

4 large avocados

MEAT/FISH

4 pounds of fresh ground meat (beef, turkey, or chicken)

8 ounces of frozen cooked shrimp

DAIRY

24 large eggs

3 35-ounce tubs of plain whole-milk Greek yogurt (such as Fage)

CANNED/ JARRED GOODS

1 12-ounce bag of organic coffee

12 ounces of green tea matcha powder

1 8-ounce jar of grass-fed ghee (clarified butter)

1 8-ounce jar of coconut oil

1 8-ounce box of baking soda

1 32-ounce bottle of apple cider vinegar

1 8-ounce bottle of coconut aminos

1 16-ounce container of sea salt

1 15-ounce jar of tomato puree

1 8-ounce can of black olives

1 8-ounce jar of hempseed oil, such as Evo Hemp

1 16-ounce jar of organic Sun-Butter

1 16-ounce jar of cashew butter

1 16-ounce jar of creamy almond butter

1 16-ounce jar of tahini

1 16-ounce jar of coconut butter (creamed coconut)

1 8-ounce jar of raw honey

1 15-ounce bottle of unsulfured blackstrap molasses

DRIED GOODS/ PANTRY ITEMS

1 17-ounce tub of protein powder (such as my Probiotic Cacao Nuzest Protein Powder)

1 17-ounce tub of pea protein powder (such as my Probiotic Vanilla Nuzest Protein Powder)

1 32-ounce tub of unflavored grass-fed gelatin, such as Vital Proteins

1 20-ounce tub of unflavored grass-fed collagen peptides, such as Vital Proteins

1 10-ounce tub of bone broth (beef or chicken)

3 pounds of unsweetened cacao powder

1 box of Evo Hemp fruit and nut bars of choice (they are the ones I recommend)

2 8-ounce boxes of chickpea or lentil pasta (gum-free, with no additives; ingredients list should just have "lentils" or "lentil flour")

1 18-ounce container of old-fashioned rolled oats

8 ounces of Evo Hemp hemp hearts

1 1-pound package of pistachio flour

One last thing: Just because a meal is listed in the menu as a "snack," that doesn't mean it can't be a meal. You can have a snack as your lunch and a dessert recipe as a snack! If you still feel hungry, eat more. If you feel full, stop. Listen to your body. We are all different, and some days you're just not as hungry as on other days. Adjust to suit how you feel. Listen to your hunger signals and honor them. You know your body best!

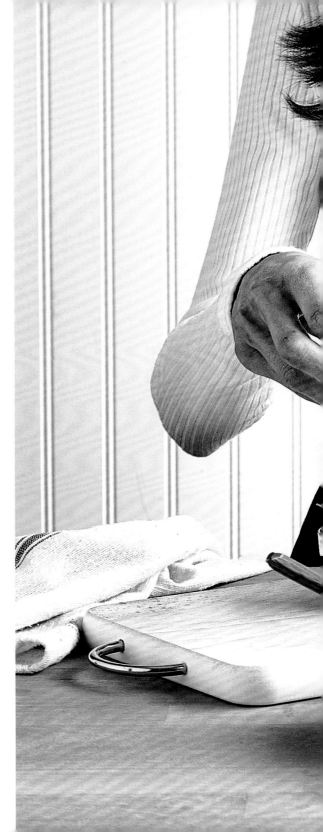

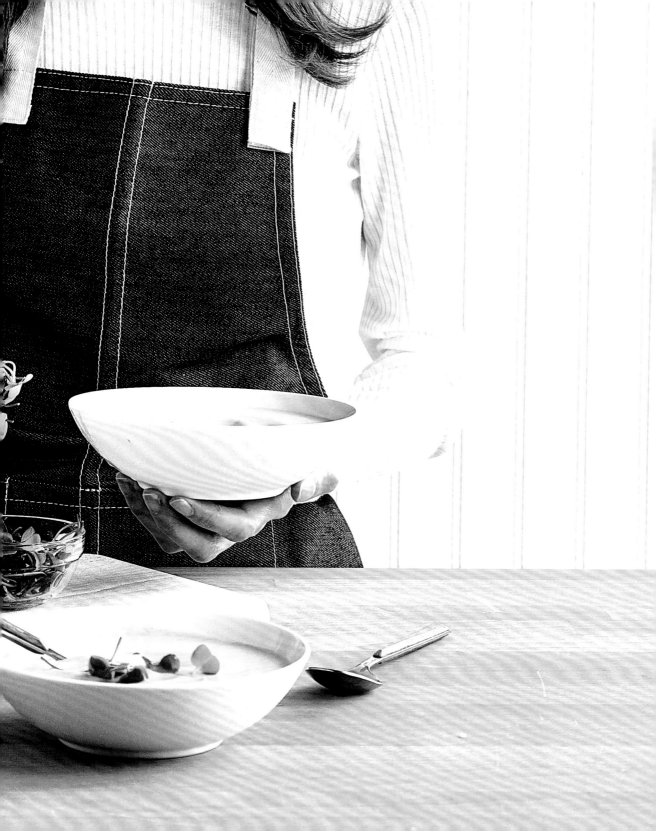

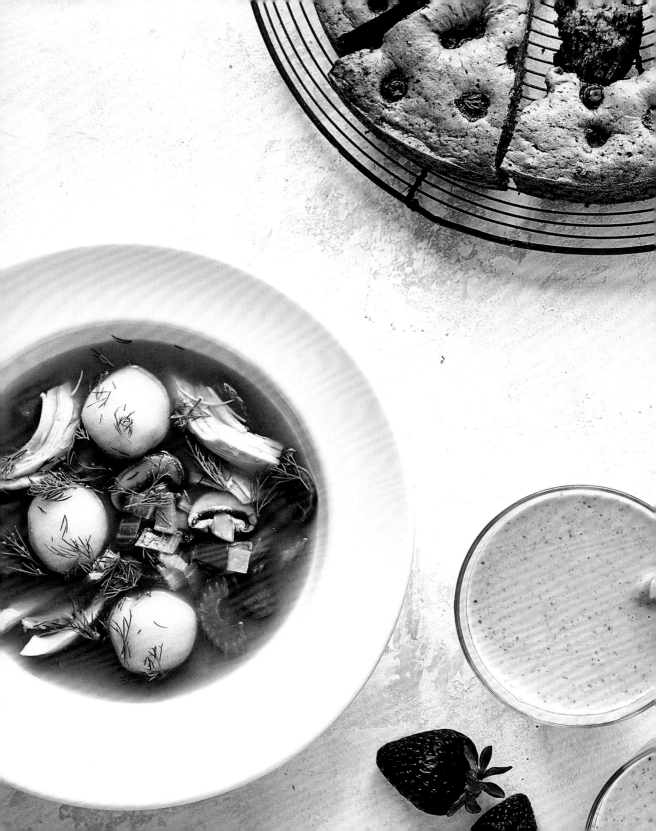

GUT-
HEALING
RECIPES

GUT RESET AND STAPLE RECIPES

Welcome to the recipes! This first recipe chapter includes the Gut Reset basics and staples that you can enjoy throughout the *Digest This* plan.

DIGESTIVE BOOST

4 whole kiwifruits, washed, skins left on

1 ripe mango, peeled, pitted, and sliced

½ ripe papaya, peeled, seeded, and sliced

½ ripe pineapple, peeled, cored, and sliced

This mixture is first on the list of staples because it *really* is a must! It helped me tremendously while healing, and it contains so many digestive benefits. No other pill, powder, or medication helped me the way this recipe did. And all I had to do was drink ½ cup of it each mid-morning! These four fruits, combined, are literally a powerhouse for optimal digestive support, containing the enzymes needed to help break down fats, carbohydrates, and proteins—and the boost is delicious, as well.

1   Place all the fruits in a blender and blend until smooth. Pour the puree into 7 individual freezer-safe cups; each serving will be about ½ cup, or 4 fluid ounces.

2   Place the cups in the freezer. Each day, remove one cup the night before, placing it in the fridge to thaw overnight.

MAKES 8 ¼-CUP SERVINGS
Prep time: 5 minutes
Cook time: 15 minutes

PUREED ANIMAL PROTEIN

8 ounces to 1 pound boneless and skinless free-range chicken or turkey breast, or already ground free-range chicken or turkey or grass-fed beef

You'll be eating pureed animal protein every day for the 21 days of the Gut Reset—and you may even want to continue this afterward, because of the great nutrient density it provides!

1   Place the breast or ground meat in a saucepan with enough water to cover. Bring the water to a boil, and then reduce the heat to low and simmer until the meat is fully cooked, about 15 minutes.

2   With a slotted spoon, transfer the meat to a blender (do not add liquid) and puree until smooth.

3   Transfer the puree to eight ¼-cup containers, cover, and store in the fridge for up to 4 days.

NOTE: You can cook the meat and let it cool before pureeing, but a tiny bit of water will be needed to facilitate the blending. Don't add too much water, or the result will be soupy.

MAKES 1 SMALL LOAF
Prep time: 10 minutes
Cook time: 30 to 35 minutes

BEST BASIC SAND- WICH BREAD

This is your go-to bread for all the sandwiches! But sandwiches are only the beginning. Try toasting it, dipping it in soup, using it for Thanksgiving stuffing, making French toast, or even crumbling it into a smoothie (yes, I've done it for an "Ice Cream Sandwich Smoothie" twist!).

1   Preheat the oven to 350°F. Grease an 8½ x 4½-inch loaf pan or line it with parchment paper.

2   With an electric or stand mixer, beat the eggs, baking soda, and vinegar until foamy and doubled in volume, about 4 minutes. Add the tahini and continue beating for 2 minutes more, until the batter is smooth and creamy.

3   Pour the batter into the prepared pan and bake for 30 to 35 minutes, or until a toothpick inserted into the center comes out clean.

4   Allow the loaf to cool briefly in the pan, then invert onto a rack to cool completely. Slice and use or store in the refrigerator for up to 5 days or in the freezer for up to 2 months.

4 large eggs

1 teaspoon baking soda

1 tablespoon apple cider vinegar

1 cup tahini

MAKES 1 SMALL LOAF
Prep time: 5 minutes
Cook time: 30 minutes

GREEN BREAD

4 large eggs

1 teaspoon baking soda

1 tablespoon apple cider vinegar

1 cup organic SunButter

Yup, *it turns green!* Why? Because the chlorogenic acid (chlorophyll) in the sunflower seeds reacts with the baking soda when baked, causing the finished product to turn green. It gradually happens during baking, but after refrigeration for a few hours, the green color really begins to show! This color is completely harmless. And, yes, it actually tastes good! The bread is perfect for St. Patrick's Day, Halloween, and even Christmas (with red jam). But don't let the holidays be the only time you make this loaf—it's delicious all year long!

1   Preheat the oven to 350°F. Grease an 8½ x 4½-inch loaf pan or line with parchment paper.

2   Whisk the eggs, baking soda, and vinegar in an electric mixer until foamy and doubled in volume. Add the SunButter and continue mixing until the batter is smooth.

3   Pour the batter into the prepared pan and bake for about 30 minutes, or until a toothpick inserted in the center comes out clean.

4   Remove from oven and let cool briefly in the pan, then invert onto a rack to cool completely. Slice and use or store in the refrigerator for up to 4 days or freeze for up to 2 weeks.

NOTE: The green color becomes deeper after 24 hours of sitting in the fridge after baking!

MAKES 6 BISCUITS
Prep time: 5 minutes
Cook time: 20 to 25 minutes

BASIC BISCUITS

4 large eggs

1 teaspoon baking soda

2 cups blanched almond flour

Go sweet! Go savory! These biscuits are the perfect blank canvas for creating endless possibilities. When I'm in the mood for something sweet, I like to add some raw honey with a little bit of SunButter, for the perfect snack. And when I'm in the mood for a savory pick-me-up, a few slices of avocado with a sprinkle of simple sea salt makes the perfect bite. These are even better as an accompaniment to warm soup, and are a crowd pleaser for entertaining during the holidays!

1 Preheat the oven to 350°F. Grease a 6-cup muffin tin or line the cups with parchment paper.

2 Whisk the eggs and baking soda in an electric mixer until foamy and doubled in volume. Gradually add the almond flour and continue mixing until the batter is smooth, about 1 minute more.

3 Pour the batter into the prepared muffin tin and bake for 20 to 25 minutes, or until a toothpick comes out clean.

4 Let the muffins cool briefly in the tin, and then invert onto a rack to cool completely. Store in the refrigerator for up to 4 days or freeze for up to 2 weeks.

MAKES 3 TO 4 CUPS
Prep time: 20 minutes
Freeze time: 4 hours

CAULI-FLOWER "CHEESE"

This is a staple, for sure! Finally, a 100 percent dairy-free cheese alternative without nutritional yeast. This melts, slices, and shreds just like cheese, too. Try the "cheddar" version grated over some chili or in a taco, or the "mozzarella" version sliced in a sandwich or as a base for pizza. I often just cut it into cubes to snack on, and I even toss the cubes into a cold pasta salad. Get creative and see what you can do!

"CHEDDAR" VERSION

1 medium head of cauliflower

1 tablespoon coconut oil, melted (or grass-fed ghee)

1 tablespoon cashew butter

1 tablespoon apple cider vinegar

1 teaspoon ground turmeric

1 teaspoon sea salt

2 teaspoons curry powder

½ tablespoon yellow mustard

4 scoops (40 grams) grass-fed gelatin of choice (such as Vital Proteins)

"MOZZARELLA" VERSION

1 medium head of cauliflower

1 tablespoon coconut oil, melted

1 tablespoon cashew butter

½ teaspoon ground white pepper

4 scoops (40 grams) unflavored grass-fed gelatin of choice (such as Vital Proteins)

1   For either version, steam the cauliflower until soft, about 5 to 10 minutes. While it is still hot or warm, puree the cauliflower in a high-speed blender (such as a Vitamix) until creamy. Do not add any liquid.

2   Add the remaining ingredients, except the gelatin, for whichever version and puree again until smooth.

3   Add the gelatin and puree one last time, making sure all the ingredients are incorporated well.

4   Pour the puree into a container lined with wax paper or parchment paper (or pour into silicone molds for cheese cubes). Refrigerate at least 4 hours, or until firm. Store in the refrigerator for no more than 5 days.

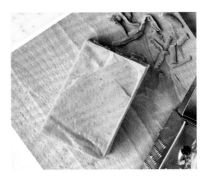

MAKES 1 CUP
Prep time: 5 minutes
Culture time: 2 to 3 days

HOME-MADE CULTURED "CREAM CHEESE"

Who knew making cream cheese could really be this easy? All you need is one prep item—a nut milk bag—and a little patience. I actually think it's fun to watch the process! My version is loaded with probiotics and protein, and actually tastes like cream cheese!

2 cups plain whole-milk cultured Greek yogurt

1 Place the yogurt in a nut milk bag (cheesecloth can also be used but is not recommended) and insert the bag into a tall, wide glass. Place a rubber band holding the bag around the top of the glass so the bag is suspended and does not touch the bottom of the glass. Place in the refrigerator overnight.

2 The next day, check the glass. You should see liquid at the bottom. Undo the rubber band and squeeze as much liquid as you can from the bag, then secure the bag again with the rubber band and refrigerate another 24 hours, allowing the yogurt to strain completely, always being sure no liquid touches the yogurt bag. This straining may be done for 2 to 3 days. At the end of the 3 days, you will have a thick, creamy spread.

3 Transfer the spread to a Tupperware or glass container and store in the refrigerator.

NOTE: Be sure to check the "use by" date on the lid of the yogurt before using and keep in mind for determining how long the spread will keep.

MAKES ABOUT 1 POUND
Prep time: 10 minutes
Chill time: 2 hours

NOFU HEMP "TOFU"

2 cups hemp seeds
(preferably Evo Hemp)

1 cup room temperature water

Juice of ½ lemon

1 teaspoon sea salt

1 to 2 teaspoons white pepper
(optional)

2 scoops (20 grams) unflavored
grass-fed gelatin of choice
(such as Vital Proteins)

Have no fear—NoFu is here! This soy-free, gum-free, even nut-free tofu alternative gets its protein and gut-healing anti-inflammatory benefits from the hemp and gelatin. There's no denying this soy swap is a winner! It's perfect on top of salads! Just be sure to keep it cold (no grilling)—it will lose its shape if heated, as the gelatin is what makes it firm (similar to the Cauliflower "Cheese" on page 106).

1   Place the hemp seeds, water, lemon juice, salt, and white pepper (if using) in a blender and puree until creamy and smooth. Taste and adjust the seasonings to taste.

2   Add the gelatin and blend again, until smooth.

3   Pour the puree into a dish lined with wax paper or parchment paper and refrigerate at least 2 hours, or until firm to the touch. Store in the fridge for up to 5 days or freeze for up to 3 weeks.

MAKES ABOUT 1 POUND
Prep time: 5 minutes
Chill time: 4 hours

HOME-MADE LUNCH MEAT

Ever just want a slice of chicken? Or a sliver of turkey? Sure, you can just snack on chicken from the bone, but there's one thing I've learned when eating healthy: You can't let yourself get bored! Taste, texture, even the look of something needs to be switched up, otherwise you "fall off the wagon" and give in to something that can really cause some tummy upsets. That's where these luncheon meat slices come into play. They're super fun layered in a sandwich, perfect for a midday snack—and you might even get your picky kids to eat meat this way. Give it a go!

2 small boneless and skinless chicken breasts, poached and cooled

½ cup almost-boiling water

2½ scoops (25 grams) unflavored grass-fed gelatin of choice (such as Vital Proteins)

2 teaspoons ground white pepper (optional)

1   Place the chicken and water in a blender and blend until smooth and creamy.

2   Add the gelatin and white pepper (if using) and blend again.

3   Wash and dry a saved BPA-free–lined 16-ounce can and transfer the chicken puree to the can. Gently tap the can on the counter to release any air bubbles. Cover and refrigerate the can for at least 4 hours, or overnight.

4   Once the chicken has firmed up, turn the can upside down onto a plate and open the other end with a can opener. You may need to squeeze the sides of the can to loosen the chicken from the sides of the mold.

5   Carefully push out the chicken loaf and slice as desired. Use the slices cold (that is, don't make a hot sandwich or warm in the oven). The loaf can be stored in the refrigerator for up to 4 days.

SMOOTHIE RECIPES FOR THE GUT RESET —AND BEYOND

What's easier to make than a smoothie? Not much! These *Digest This* smoothies were developed to meet the Gut Reset guidelines, so you can choose any of them during the 21-day Gut Reset. They're so delicious, though, you'll want to enjoy them any time!

Each recipe makes 1 serving.

Note that when it comes to gelatin and collagen protein, pea protein, and other proteins (like my Probiotic Cacao Nuzest Protein Powder), the sizes of scoops may vary, depending on the brand, and this affects the serving size somewhat. To help clarify, I've indicated gram equivalencies for the scoop measurements, such as "1 scoop (10 grams)" or for standard amounts like ¼ cup.

SWEET POTATO-CHOCOLATE CHERRY

smoothie

½ cup plain whole-milk cultured Greek yogurt

½ cup frozen cooked sweet potato cubes (about 1 inch)

¼ cup frozen cherries

1 cup frozen cooked cauliflower florets

3 ice cubes

1 tablespoon unsweetened cocoa powder

2 scoops (20 grams) unflavored grass-fed collagen of choice (such as Vital Proteins)

This smoothie is so thick that I always want to call it ice cream. And who could turn down ice cream for a meal? I mean, if it's healthy and loaded with nutrients that are good for the gut, why pass it up? Adding sweet potatoes to your smoothies will lend a creaminess, natural sweetness, B and C vitamins, and a load of beta-carotene. This smoothie is one you'll be making often, for more reasons than one!

Place all the ingredients in a high-speed blender in the order listed. Gradually increase the blender speed and use a tamper (if available) to push down so as to mix all the ingredients until smooth. (Or, stop the blender periodically and scrape down the sides.) Pour into a glass and enjoy.

BUTTERNUT APPLE PIE
smoothie

Imagine a slice of warm apple pie with a scoop of creamy vanilla ice cream on top! This is basically all those flavors in one thick, luscious smoothie. Thankfully, apples and butternut squash are available year-round, so you have no excuse for not making this any time you crave apple pie.

Place all the ingredients in a high-speed blender in the order listed. Gradually increase the blender speed and use a tamper (if available) to push down so as to mix the ingredients until smooth. (Or, stop the blender periodically and scrape down the sides.) Pour into a glass and enjoy.

½ cup plain whole-milk cultured Greek yogurt

1 cup frozen cooked butternut squash cubes (about 1 inch)

½ cup frozen chopped apple

1 tablespoon almond butter

3 ice cubes

2 scoops (20 grams) unflavored grass-fed collagen of choice (such as Vital Proteins)

½ teaspoon ground cinnamon

BEET THE BLUES

smoothie

½ cup plain whole-milk cultured Greek yogurt

½ cup frozen wild blueberries

¼ cup frozen chopped cooked beets

1 cup frozen cooked cauliflower florets

1 tablespoon cashew butter

3 ice cubes

2 scoops (20 grams) unflavored grass-fed collagen of choice (such as Vital Proteins)

Okay, I couldn't resist these puns, for this deep, rich smoothie! But in all seriousness, beets and blueberries are a must-try in a smoothie. Don't let the colors intimidate you—instead, embrace them. This is an antioxidant powerhouse sure to lift anyone's mood!

Place all the ingredients in a high-speed blender in the order listed. Gradually increase the blender speed and use a tamper (if available) to push down so as to mix the ingredients until smooth. (Or, stop the blender periodically and scrape down the sides.) Pour into a glass and enjoy.

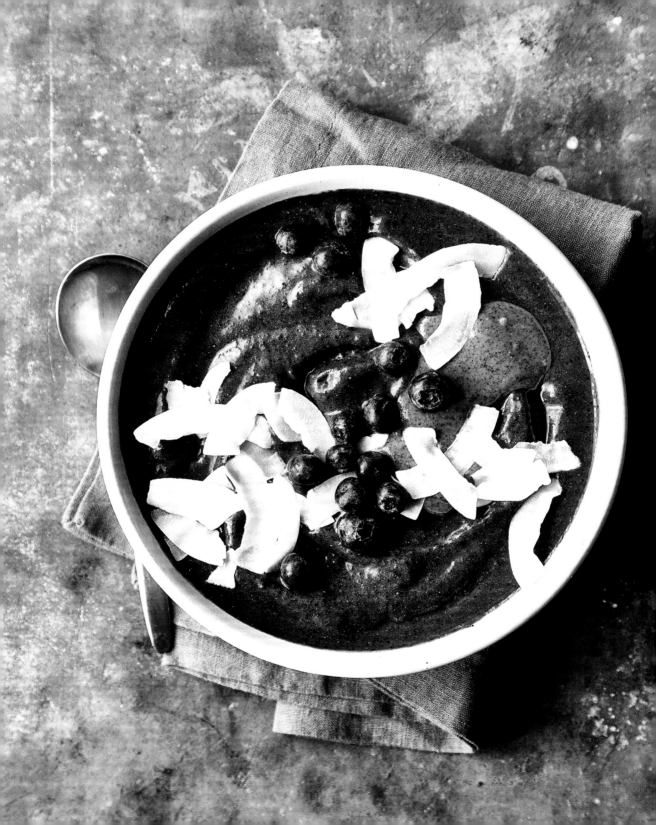

FRENCH VANILLA "MILKSHAKE"

½ cup plain whole-milk cultured Greek yogurt

1 cup frozen cooked cauliflower florets

¾ cup frozen cooked white sweet potato cubes (about 1 inch)

1 tablespoon cashew butter (optional; added for blending or on top afterward)

3 ice cubes

Pinch of minced vanilla bean

2 scoops (20 grams) unflavored grass-fed collagen of choice (such as Vital Proteins)

You really can't go wrong with vanilla! It's a classic flavor that almost everyone agrees on. What makes this smoothie resemble a vanilla milkshake is the white sweet potato (found in most grocery stores). The white sweet potatoes really do taste like vanilla! Plus, with cashew butter and the vanilla collagen, this shake is on vanilla overload! It's honestly one of my favorites!

Place all the ingredients in a high-speed blender in the order listed. Gradually increase the blender speed and use a tamper (if available) to push down so as to mix the ingredients until smooth. (Or, stop the blender periodically and scrape down the sides.) Pour into a glass and enjoy.

HEALTHIEST CHOCOLATE "FROSTY"

Could this possibly be the *healthiest* chocolate "frosty" ever? I may be biased, but I think so! Where else can you order a frosty made from squash and cauliflower, which is loaded with probiotics and protein, full of gut-healing properties, and with no refined sugar—and that actually tastes like dessert? You can't turn down this creamy treat. I mean, lunch. Or dinner!

Place all the ingredients in a high-speed blender in the order listed. Gradually increase the blender speed and use a tamper (if available) to push down so as to mix ingredients until smooth. (Or, stop the blender periodically and scrape down the sides.) Pour into a glass and enjoy.

½ cup plain whole-milk cultured Greek yogurt

1 cup frozen cooked cauliflower florets

¾ cup frozen cooked butternut squash cubes (about 1 inch)

1 tablespoon organic SunButter (or nut or seed butter of choice)

1 tablespoon date syrup or unsulfured blackstrap molasses

1 tablespoon unsweetened cocoa powder

3 ice cubes

2 scoops (20 grams) chocolate protein powder of choice (such as my Probiotic Cacao Nuzest Protein Powder)

STRAW-BERRIES 'N' CREAM
smoothie

½ cup plain whole-milk cultured Greek yogurt

1 cup frozen chopped peeled cucumber

½ cup frozen cooked white sweet potato cubes (about 1 inch)

½ cup frozen sliced strawberries

1 tablespoon cashew butter (optional; added for blending or on top afterward)

3 ice cubes

2 scoops (20 grams) unflavored grass-fed collagen of choice (such as Vital Proteins)

Remember those Strawberries 'n' Cream hard candies with the pink and white swirls? I used to eat those by the bag as a kid. (Please don't do that!) This smoothie reminds me of those and brings me back to my childhood. You may not realize strawberries are actually pretty low in sugar compared to other fruits (just 8 grams per 1 cup), but they still provide a sweetness we all know and love! Feel free to add some unsweetened chocolate chips after blending for a "chocolate strawberry" version, or leave this just as is for the perfectly balanced meal that tastes like dessert.

Place all the ingredients in a high-speed blender in the order listed. Gradually increase the blender speed and use a tamper (if available) to push down so as to mix the ingredients until smooth. (Or, stop the blender periodically and scrape down the sides.) Pour into a glass and enjoy.

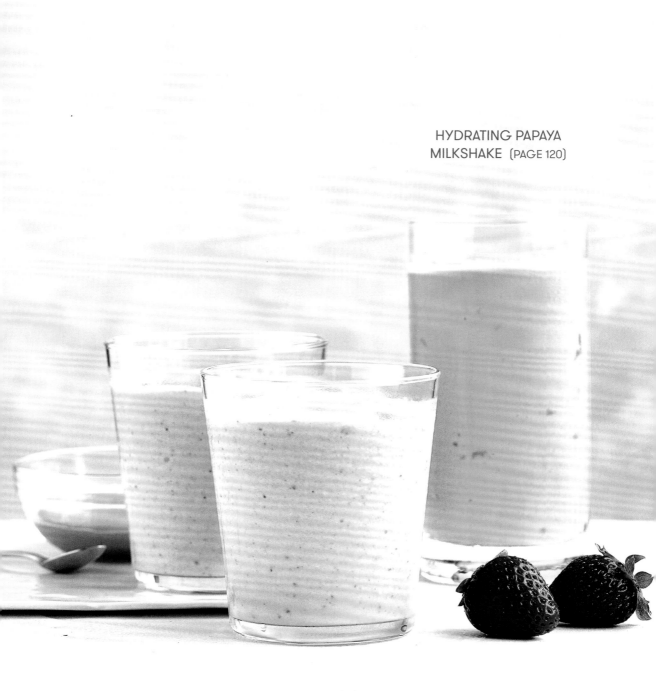

HYDRATING PAPAYA
MILKSHAKE (PAGE 120)

STRAWBERRIES 'N' CREAM
SMOOTHIE

HYDRATING PAPAYA MILK-SHAKE

½ cup plain whole-milk cultured Greek yogurt

1 cup frozen chopped peeled cucumber

1 cup frozen chopped papaya

1 tablespoon cashew butter (optional; added for blending or on top afterward)

3 ice cubes

2 scoops (20 grams) unflavored grass-fed collagen of choice (such as Vital Proteins)

Cucumber is 95 percent water, which means including it in smoothies is ideal for hydration! Plus, cucumbers can't really "melt" (like ice does), so they won't water down your smoothie! With the combination of moist cucumber, digestive papaya, probiotic Greek yogurt, and the collagen, this recipe is as easy as pie—or a milkshake! (See photo on page 119)

Place all the ingredients in a high-speed blender in the order listed. Gradually increase the blender speed and use a tamper (if available) to push down so as to mix the ingredients. (Or, stop the blender periodically and scrape down the sides.) Pour into a glass and enjoy.

MINT 'N' CHOCOLATE CHIP HEMP
smoothie

Okay, I know I say every smoothie is my favorite recipe—but this has to be up there at the top of the list! Perhaps it's because mint chocolate chip was one of my favorite ice creams as a kid. I would always choose this flavor on those late-night runs to the drugstore, where they served it up by the scoop. Who knew all along I loved a flavor that actually helps with bloating and gas? (See photo on page 122)

Place all the ingredients in a high-speed blender in the order listed. Gradually increase the blender speed and use a tamper (if available) to push down so as to mix the ingredients until smooth. (Or, stop the blender periodically and scrape down the sides.) Pour into a glass and enjoy.

½ cup plain whole-milk cultured Greek yogurt

1 cup frozen chopped peeled cucumber

½ cup frozen cooked butternut squash cubes (about 1 inch)

1 Medjool date, pitted

Sprig of fresh mint

Handful of unsweetened chocolate chips

1 tablespoon unsweetened cocoa powder

3 ice cubes

¼ cup (30 grams) protein powder of choice (such as Evo Hemp Pro 90)

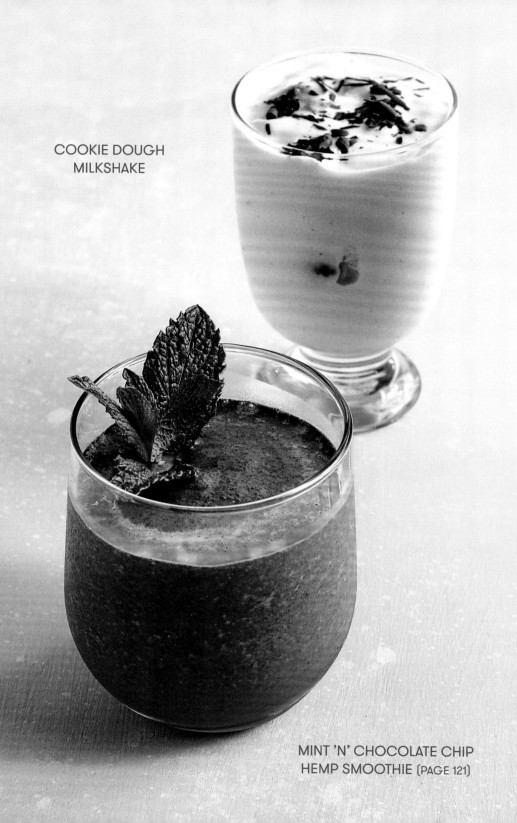

COOKIE DOUGH
MILKSHAKE

MINT 'N' CHOCOLATE CHIP
HEMP SMOOTHIE (PAGE 121)

COOKIE DOUGH MILK-SHAKE

Better than cookie dough ice cream? I think so! After all, does the average cookie dough ice cream contain probiotics? Does the average cookie dough ice cream contain protein? Does the average cookie dough ice cream contain essential nutrients and gut healing properties? These are just a few reasons why this recipe is ten times better than the average! But what's the best part? It actually tastes good!

Place all the ingredients (except the dough bites) in a high-speed blender in the order listed. Gradually increase the blender speed and use a tamper (if available) to push down so as to mix the ingredients until smooth. (Or, stop the blender periodically and scrape down the sides.) Pour into a glass, add the dough bites, and enjoy!

½ cup plain whole-milk cultured Greek yogurt

1 cup frozen cooked cauliflower florets

½ cup frozen cooked white sweet potato cubes (about 1 inch)

1 tablespoon organic SunButter (or nut or seed butter of choice)

Pinch of minced vanilla bean

3 ice cubes

2 scoops (20 grams) unflavored grass-fed collagen of choice (such as Vital Proteins)

3 Easy-Peasy Protein Cookie Dough Bites (page 210)

PUMPKIN PIE SHAKE

½ cup plain whole-milk cultured Greek yogurt

1 cup frozen peeled and chopped uncooked zucchini

½ cup frozen cooked pumpkin cubes (about 1 inch)

1 tablespoon organic SunButter (or nut or seed butter of choice)

3 ice cubes

2 scoops (20 grams) chocolate protein powder of choice (such as my Probiotic Cacao Nuzest Protein Powder)

½ teaspoon pumpkin pie spice

1 Medjool date, pitted

Pumpkin pie is great any time of the year! Of course, fresh baking pumpkins are only available in the fall and winter months, so take advantage of that and enjoy this while you can. You can also prepare extra amounts of pumpkin and freeze them to last you long into the new year.

Place all the ingredients in a high-speed blender in the order listed. Gradually increase the blender speed and use a tamper (if available) to push down so as to mix the ingredients until smooth. (Or, stop the blender periodically and scrape down the sides.) Pour into a glass and enjoy.

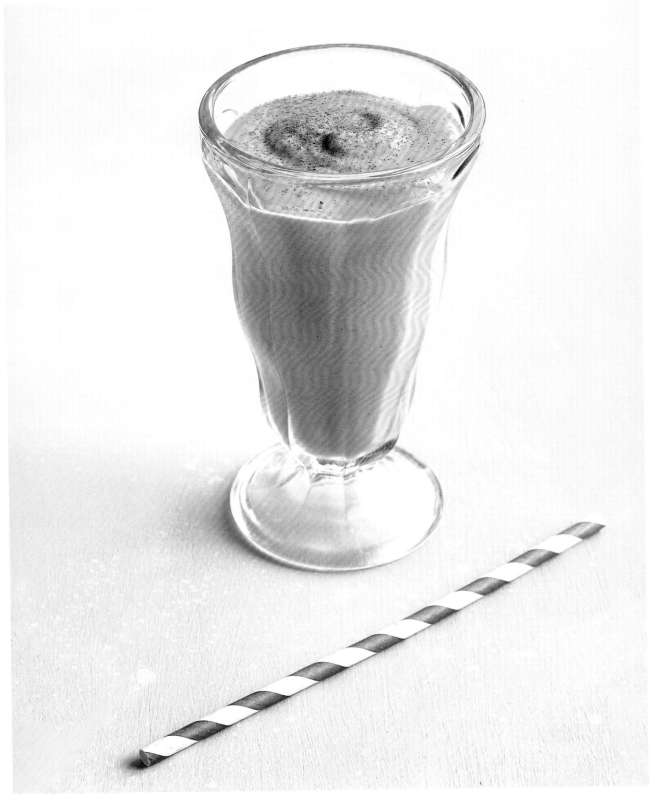

"PB&J" SAND-WICH
smoothie

½ cup plain whole-milk cultured Greek yogurt

1 cup frozen cooked cauliflower florets

¾ cup frozen cooked white sweet potato cubes (about 1 inch)

Handful of frozen halved strawberries (or other berry of choice)

1 tablespoon organic SunButter (optional; add at blending or on top afterward)

3 ice cubes

2 scoops (20 grams) unflavored grass-fed collagen of choice (such as Vital Proteins)

1–2 tablespoons crumbled Best Basic Sandwich Bread (page 103), for topping

This peanut butter–less PB&J smoothie takes me back to my home-school days, when all I ever ate was this classic sandwich. Now as an adult, I still have that craving and have no shame in saying so! What better way to transform a childhood favorite into a more sophisticated smoothie full of gut-healing benefits?

Place all the ingredients (except the topping) in a high-speed blender in the order listed. Gradually increase the blender speed and use a tamper (if available) to push down so as to mix the ingredients until smooth. (Or, stop the blender periodically and scrape down the sides.) Pour the smoothie into a glass. Top with the crumbled bread and enjoy.

BANANA BREAD
smoothie

Banana bread—in smoothie form? Yes, please! I used to hate bananas (we all have those phases, right?), but over time I learned to love them. So, if you're one of those who aren't on Team Banana, give this a try anyway. You may surprise yourself and change your team. And if you're already a banana bread lover, then I don't think you need any convincing to make this smoothie!

Place all the ingredients (except the topping) in a high-speed blender in the order listed. Gradually increase the blender speed and use a tamper (if available) to push down so as to mix the ingredients until smooth. (Or, stop the blender periodically and scrape down the sides.) Pour the smoothie into a glass. Top with the crumbled bread.

½ cup plain, whole-milk cultured Greek yogurt

1 frozen peeled banana

¾ cup frozen chopped peeled cucumber

1 tablespoon organic SunButter (or other nut or seed butter of choice)

2 tablespoons raisins (optional)

2 scoops (20 grams) unflavored grass-fed collagen of choice (such as Vital Proteins)

1–2 tablespoons crumbled Best Basic Sandwich Bread (page 103), for topping

FRUIT-FREE "FROSTY"

½ cup plain whole-milk cultured Greek yogurt

1 cup frozen chopped peeled cucumber

½ cup frozen cooked white sweet potato cubes (about 1 inch)

½ cup frozen cooked butternut squash cubes (about 1 inch)

1 tablespoon unsweetened cocoa powder

Splash of water or nut milk

2 scoops (20 grams) chocolate protein powder of choice (such as my Probiotic Cacao Nuzest Protein Powder)

Fruit-free? Why? There's certainly nothing wrong with fruit, but even so, we can all overdo it on the fruit sugar some days. This recipe is for when you're feeling you've had your limit of fruit sugar but still crave a smoothie (or need it for digestion reasons). It's not savory, but it's also not extra sweet.

Some days I make this recipe when I've eaten lunch that was on the sweeter side and I don't feel like eating dessert (okay, yes, I've had those moments). Your taste buds will soon change and you'll start noticing the natural flavors of each ingredient. And when you do get to that point, you'll also notice the white sweet potato and butternut squash in this recipe, with their sweet notes!

Place all the ingredients in a high-speed blender in the order listed. Gradually increase the blender speed and use a tamper (if available) to push down so as to mix the ingredients until smooth. (Or, stop the blender periodically and scrape down the sides.) Pour into a glass and enjoy.

DOUBLE FUDGE "FROSTY"

What's better than a fudge frosty? Answer: a Double Fudge "Frosty"! Double the fudge, double the fun! This combo will please literally anyone. The creaminess of the sweet potato sends it over the top. Plus, it's high in iron from the black-strap molasses. This is a double win!

Place all the ingredients in a high-speed blender in the order listed. Gradually increase the blender speed and use a tamper (if available) to push down so as to mix the ingredients until smooth. (Or, stop the blender periodically and scrape down the sides.) Pour into a glass and enjoy.

½ cup plain whole-milk cultured Greek yogurt

1 cup frozen peeled chopped uncooked zucchini

½ cup frozen cooked sweet potato cubes (about 1 inch)

1 tablespoon unsulfured blackstrap molasses

2 tablespoons unsweetened cocoa powder

3 ice cubes

2 scoops (20 grams) chocolate protein powder of choice (such as my Probiotic Cacao Nuzest Protein Powder)

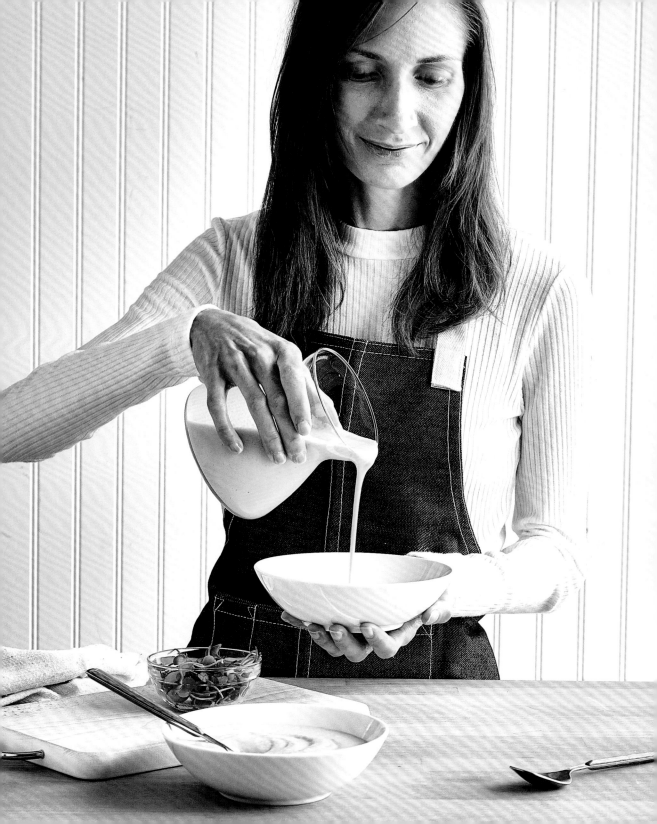

SWEET PEA GAZPA- CHO

This smoothie is more on the savory side, and more of a chilled soup—perfect for those hot summer nights when you want something fresh and light! The cucumbers are super hydrating and soothing to the gut. Paired with Greek yogurt for added protein and probiotics, and avocado for healthy fat, this combo gives you the creaminess you've always wanted in a gazpacho.

Place all the ingredients in a high-speed blender in the order listed. Gradually increase the blender speed and use a tamper (if available) to push down so as to mix the ingredients until smooth. (Or, stop the blender periodically and scrape down the sides.) Pour into a glass and enjoy.

½ cup plain whole-milk cultured Greek yogurt

1 cup frozen chopped peeled cucumber

½ cup frozen sweet peas

½ small avocado, peeled and pitted

3 ice cubes

2 scoops (20 grams) unflavored grass-fed collagen of choice (such as Vital Proteins)

COOKIES 'N' CREAM HEMP SHAKE

½ cup plain whole-milk cultured
Greek yogurt

1 cup frozen cooked
cauliflower florets

½ cup frozen cooked white sweet
potato cubes (about 1 inch)

1 tablespoon coconut butter
(creamed coconut), melted

1 tablespoon hemp seeds of choice
(such as Evo Hemp)

¼ teaspoon minced vanilla bean

3 ice cubes

¼ cup hemp protein powder of
choice (such as Evo Hemp Pro 90)

¼ cup crumbled Probiotic Vegan
Brownies (page 234)

If I had to choose, cookies 'n' cream has to be one of my all-time favorite shake combos! I could eat this over and over again (and I have!) without getting tired of it. And because it's the healthy version, you won't have any guilt or digestive upsets if you did, too. It's basically like Oreos mixed in a creamy vanilla bean ice cream. I mean, who can say no to that?!

Place all the ingredients (except the brownie crumbs) in a high-speed blender in the order listed. Gradually increase the blender speed and use a tamper (if available) to push down so as to mix the ingredients until smooth. (Or, stop the blender periodically and scrape down the sides.) Pour into a glass. Stir in the brownie crumbs and enjoy!

CHERRY CHOCOLATE CHIP MILKSHAKE

Cherries and chocolate were just meant to be! Agreed? Here's a fun fact about cherries: Studies show that they are one of the few foods naturally containing melatonin, the chemical that helps regulate sleep and calmness. So, eating a cherry-based meal at night may give you just what you need for a good night's rest!

Place all the ingredients in a high-speed blender in the order listed. Gradually increase the blender speed and use a tamper (if available) to push down so as to mix the ingredients until smooth. (Or, stop the blender periodically and scrape down the sides.) Pour into a glass and enjoy.

½ cup plain whole-milk cultured Greek yogurt

1 cup frozen cooked cauliflower florets

½ cup frozen cooked butternut squash cubes (about 1 inch)

8 frozen pitted dark cherries

1 tablespoon unsweetened chocolate chips

1 tablespoon unsweetened cocoa powder

3 ice cubes

2 scoops (20 grams) chocolate protein powder of choice (such as my Probiotic Cacao Nuzest Protein Powder)

BREAK-
FAST
RECIPES

Your mom was right about breakfast being the most important meal of the day. I have Gut-Healing Frothy Coffee (page 216) just about every morning, but when it comes to breakfast, sometimes I want something sweet (like doughnuts—yum!), while other mornings, something more savory hits the spot.

MAKES 1 SERVING
Prep time: 5 minutes
Chill time: 12 hours

SOAKED CHOCOLATE PROBIOTIC OATMEAL

Soaking oats is similar to sprouting them, and it reduces the phytic acid, which can cause stomach upset and malabsorption of nutrients. So, if you've always felt that oatmeal or oats in general never really "agreed" with you, or you've always had a difficult time digesting them, try soaking! Just make sure to include a squeeze of fresh lemon juice to neutralize the phytic acid in the bowl—this way you don't even have to drain them! I prefer the taste of cold oats to the hot stove top variety, and personally I think they taste like cake batter (and who doesn't want cake batter for breakfast?).

½ cup old-fashioned rolled oats

1 tablespoon fresh lemon juice

1 cup filtered water

1 scoop (12.5 grams) chocolate protein powder of choice (such as my Probiotic Cacao Nuzest Protein Powder)

1 tablespoon unsweetened cocoa powder

1 In a bowl, mix all the ingredients well and refrigerate overnight.

2 Remove the bowl from the refrigerator the next morning, stir well, then add the desired toppings and enjoy.

OPTIONAL TOPPINGS

Raw honey

Sprouted nuts or seeds

Unsweetened chocolate chips or cacao nibs

MAKES 8 PULL-APART SCONES
Prep time: 10 minutes
Cook time: 20 minutes

BLUE-BERRY PROTEIN SCONES

Imagine waking up to freshly baked blueberry scones. Now stop imagining that and make 'em! Breakfast just might become your favorite meal of the day (if it isn't already) after making these tasty buns loaded with gut-healthy protein, a dash of healthy fat, and lightly sweetened with coconut sugar (totally optional, if you want to leave it out). They're even kid-approved!

4 large eggs

1 teaspoon baking soda

2 tablespoons fresh lemon juice

½ cup creamy cashew butter

½ cup coconut sugar

3 scoops (30 grams) pea protein powder of choice (such as Probiotic Vanilla Nuzest Protein Powder)

½ cup frozen wild blueberries

1 Preheat the oven to 350°F. Line an 8-inch round baking pan with parchment paper.

2 Mix all the ingredients except the blueberries in a bowl. Pour the batter into the prepared pan. Drop the blueberries evenly on top, and bake for about 20 minutes or until a toothpick inserted in the center comes out clean.

3 Let the pan cool completely on a rack. Slice into squares and serve. Store in the refrigerator for up to 3 days or freeze for up to 2 weeks.

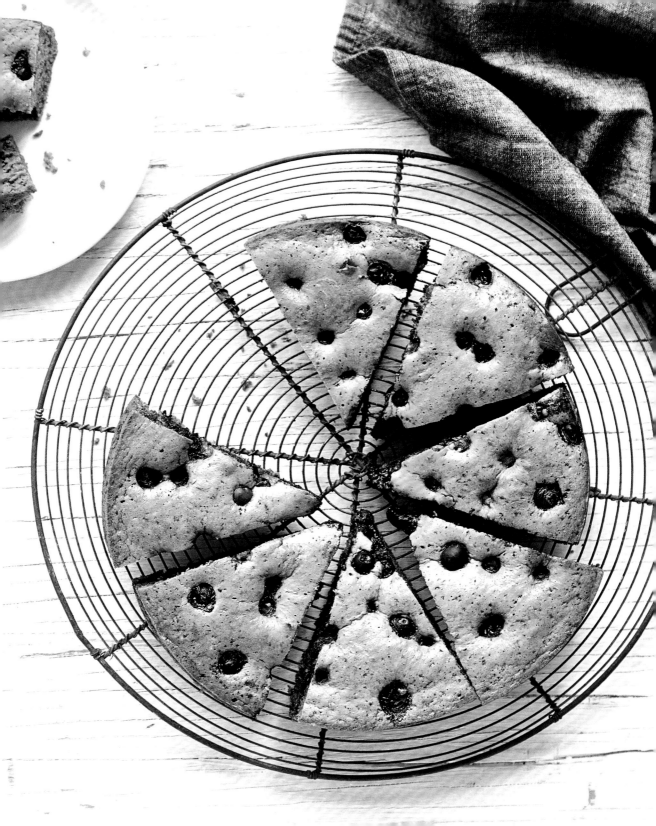

MAKES 8 SERVINGS
Prep time: 10 minutes
Cook time: 20 minutes

MACA MOCHA COFFEE CAKE

1 teaspoon baking soda

4 large eggs

½ cup creamy almond butter

3 scoops (37.5 grams) chocolate protein powder of choice (such as my Probiotic Cacao Nuzest Protein Powder)

3 tablespoons unsweetened cocoa powder

½ teaspoon instant coffee, plus extra to sprinkle on top

2 teaspoons maca powder

1 teaspoon ground cinnamon

¼ cup coconut sugar

OPTIONAL TOPPINGS

Extra almond butter

Unsweetened coconut butter (creamed coconut)

If you don't know me by now, know this: I love coffee! I always start my day with my Gut-Healing Frothy Coffee (page 216), but if I can have a healthy cake flavored like a cup of joe, then you know I'm 100 percent for it! I mean, who can resist a good slice of coffee cake?

1   Preheat the oven to 350°F. Line an 8-inch baking pan with parchment paper.

2   Whip all the ingredients together in a bowl and pour into the prepared pan. Sprinkle the top with a bit more coffee and swirl with a toothpick. Bake for 20 minutes, or until a toothpick inserted in the center comes out clean.

3   Allow the cake to cool in the pan, then drizzle with the optional toppings, cut into serving squares, and serve. Store in the refrigerator for up to 4 days or freeze for up to 2 weeks.

MAKES 2 SERVINGS
Prep time: 15 minutes
Cook time: 15 to 20 minutes

COCOA COLL- AGEN PUFF CEREAL

Growing up, I ate cold cereal every single day. We never had pancakes or waffles, and had eggs only on special occasions. So, cold cereal really has a special place in my heart and brings me back to my childhood days. Of course, most cereals today contain many additives and gut irritants, and are loaded with refined sugar. Thankfully, my mind has no limits, and if I want something, I'll make it happen! Like these healthified Cocoa Collagen Puffs!

1 Preheat the oven to 300°F. Line a baking sheet with parchment paper.

2 Melt the coconut oil in a small saucepan over low heat along with the maple syrup, nut or seed butter, cinnamon, and cocoa powder until it forms a sauce, a few minutes. Stir in the collagen.

3 Place the puffed rice cereal in a bowl and pour on the sauce. Stir to coat, then spread out on the baking sheet.

4 Bake for 15 to 20 minutes, moving the rice cereal around with a spoon halfway through baking, until the puffed rice is light brown in color. Allow to cool completely; cooling makes the puffed rice crispy. Store in an airtight container for up to 2 days at room temperature.

1 teaspoon coconut oil

3 tablespoons pure maple syrup

1½ tablespoons nut or seed butter, such as organic SunButter

1 teaspoon ground cinnamon

3 tablespoons unsweetened cocoa powder

2 scoops (20 grams) unflavored grass-fed collagen of choice (such as Vital Proteins)

2 cups puffed brown rice cereal (with no added ingredients)

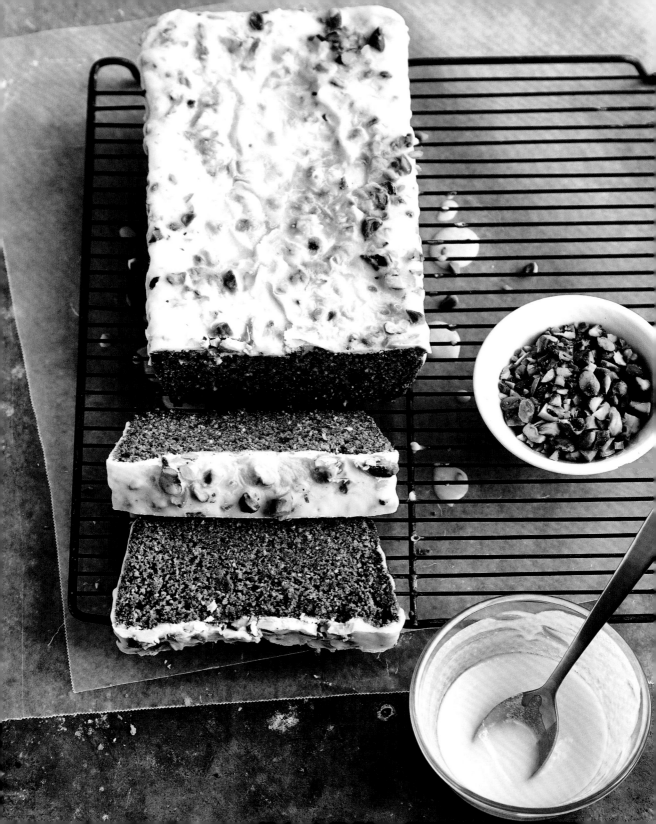

MAKES 8 SERVINGS
Prep time: 10 minutes
Cook time: 25 minutes

ICED PISTACHIO COCONUT CAKE

This one is for all my pistachio lovers. I'm taking you down the green path of decadent pound cake turned healthy! I love to crumble a slice and mix it into one of my smoothie recipes for the ultimate (rejuvenating) treat. And did I mention there's absolutely NO added sugar? I find pistachios have a natural sweetness to them, and with the pure coconut buttercream icing on top, you really don't need anything extra (because this is extra already).

1   Preheat the oven to 350°F. Line an 8½ x 8½-inch loaf pan with parchment paper.

2   In a large bowl, combine the baking soda and vinegar, and allow to fizz for a few minutes.

3   Add the eggs and mix with an electric or stand mixer until the eggs begin to be foamy and double in volume, 2 to 3 minutes.

4   Stir in the coconut butter, pistachio flour, and coconut flour. Continue to beat until the batter is smooth.

5   Pour the batter into the prepared pan and bake for about 25 minutes, or until a toothpick inserted in the center comes out clean. Allow the cake to cool completely (or refrigerate or, even better, freeze).

6   Drizzle the melted coconut butter over the cake and immediately sprinkle with the pistachios. If the bread is ice cold, the coconut butter will instantly harden, so be quick when topping with the pistachios. Slice and serve. Store any extra in the refrigerator for up to 4 days or freeze for up to 2 weeks.

1 teaspoon baking soda

1 tablespoon apple cider vinegar

4 large eggs

¼ cup coconut butter (creamed coconut)

2 cups pistachio flour

¼ cup coconut flour

TOPPINGS

Melted coconut butter (creamed coconut)

Raw pistachios

MAKES 21 CUBES
Prep time: 5 minutes
Chill time: 2 to 3 hours

COCO-NUT COFFEE CUBES

1 cup strong hot coffee

1 tablespoon grass-fed ghee
(clarified butter)

1 tablespoon coconut oil

3 scoops (30 grams) unflavored
grass-fed gelatin of choice
(such as Vital Proteins)

Have you ever chewed your coffee? If you haven't, I think it's about time you experienced this fun way to get that burst of energy, and without any gut upsets! This recipe is similar to my morning Gut-Healing Frothy Coffee (page 216), but it is super concentrated. That said, you need only 3 or 4 small cubes per serving. Feel free to pop a few in your mouth before the gym, enjoy a couple as an afternoon snack, or incorporate them into your morning breakfast routine! You can even drop a few in your coffee for an extra coffee kick!

Blend all the ingredients in a high-speed blender, and then pour the mixture into 1-inch silicone molds or one large dish. Refrigerate for 2 to 3 hours. Pop the cubes out of the molds or, if using the single dish, slice into squares. Store in the refrigerator for up to 5 days.

MAKES 5 LARGE BAGELS
Prep time: 10 minutes
Cook time: 20 minutes

GRAIN-FREE BONE BROTH BAGELS

Bone broth can be enjoyed in so many ways! Even in bagels! It may sound odd, but you can't even taste the broth while enjoying these fluffy *hole*-some baked goods. Try these bagels with my Homemade Cultured "Cream Cheese" (page 107) and a side of Gut-Healing Frothy Coffee (page 216), and you're ready to take on the day! Or try them with Greek yogurt and avocado, or berries, SunButter with banana, or tuna for a quick healthy meal.

1 Preheat the oven to 350°F. Grease a doughnut baking tin with at least 5 cups, or use 5 silicone molds.

2 With an electric or stand mixer, whisk the eggs and baking soda until the eggs are foamy and doubled in volume. Add the almond flour and bone broth powder, and continue mixing for 1 minute more.

3 Transfer the batter to the prepared tin and bake for about 20 minutes, or until a toothpick inserted in the center of one comes out clean. Allow to cool on a rack before popping out of the mold, then slice in half. Store in the refrigerator for up to 2 days or freeze for up to 2 weeks.

4 whole eggs

1 teaspoon baking soda

2 cups blanched almond flour

2 scoops (20 grams) chicken bone broth powder of choice (such as Vital Proteins)

BAKED BREAK- FAST OATMEAL COOKIE

1¼ cups old-fashioned rolled oats

2 tablespoons raisins

2 cups filtered water

Juice from ½ lemon

2 scoops (25 grams) chocolate protein powder of choice (such as my Probiotic Cacao Nuzest Protein Powder)

3 tablespoons unsweetened cocoa powder

OPTIONAL TOPPINGS

Unsweetened chocolate pieces

Raw honey or unsulfured blackstrap molasses

Sea salt

Unsweetened coconut butter (creamed coconut)

Cookies for breakfast? Yes, please! This is what I call "adulting." Remember, just because it's called a "cookie," that doesn't mean it's bad for your gut. It's all about what you put into the cookie and the way you prepare it. I suggest baking a bunch of these ahead of time and storing them in the refrigerator for the days to come. That way, if you find yourself in a rush the next morning, you have no excuse to skip breakfast.

1   Soak the oats and raisins in the filtered water along with the lemon juice for at least 3 hours or overnight in the refrigerator. Drain any excess water.

2   Preheat the oven to 350°F. Grease a baking dish or line a baking sheet with parchment paper.

3   Mix the soaked oats with the protein powder and cocoa powder, and spread in the prepared baking dish or on the baking sheet. Bake for about 30 minutes, or until a toothpick inserted in the center comes out clean. Top with your chosen toppings and enjoy. For leftovers, allow to cool and store in an airtight container in the refrigerator for up to 3 days, or freeze for up to 1 week.

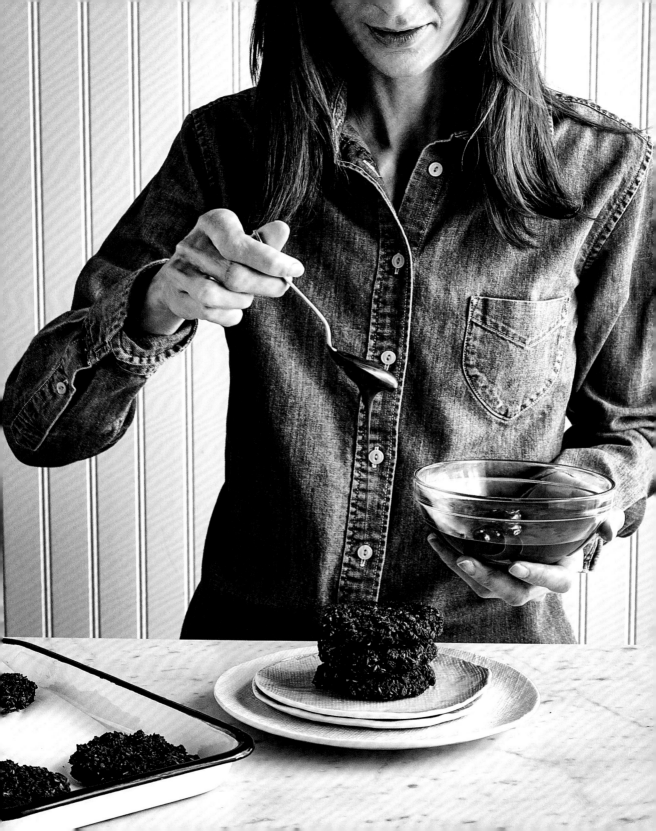

MAKES 3 TO 5 SERVINGS
Prep time: 15 minutes
Cook time: 5 minutes

SWEET POTATO HEMP TOAST

1 large sweet potato

2 large eggs

½ teaspoon baking soda

¼ cup hemp protein powder of choice (such as Evo Hemp Pro 90)

3 tablespoons cassava flour

Dash of ground cinnamon

Grass-fed ghee or coconut oil, for frying

TOPPING

Unsulfured blackstrap molasses

We've all heard of sweet potato toast, but I'm taking it to the next level with an anti-inflammatory version made as French toast! Feel free to grace it with your preferred "French toast" toppings; however, I recommend blackstrap molasses.

Have you tried blackstrap molasses? No need to fear this sweet syrup—remember, everything in moderation. And unsulfured blackstrap molasses is actually super high in iron and offers a great little boost of energy, if taken in the morning. And with the added benefits of the anti-inflammatory hemp protein powder here, you've got the perfect fuel to start your day!

1 Slice the sweet potato and toast in a toaster or toaster oven for 3 to 5 minutes, until tender.

2 In a large bowl, whisk the eggs with the baking soda; add the hemp protein, cassava flour, and cinnamon, and mix until a smooth batter forms.

3 Spray a large skillet with oil or ghee and place over medium heat. Dredge each sweet potato slice in the batter and then cook on each side for 2 to 3 minutes. Top with blackstrap molasses and enjoy.

MAKES 1 SERVING
Prep time: 5 minutes
Cook time: 10 minutes

"BANILLA" BEAN PROTEIN PANCAKE

Who knew you could make pancakes out of so few ingredients (and no flour)? These are a fun, healthy twist on a classic favorite that will bring everyone to the table Sunday morning! Add a small amount of plain carbonated water to your eggs to make the batter fluffier.

1 Whisk the banana in a bowl together with the eggs and mineral water until foamy and doubled in volume. Add the vanilla beans and collagen, and continue mixing for a smooth batter.

2 Heat a medium skillet with a drizzle of the oil, then carefully pour the batter into the skillet and cook for about 1 minute or until you start to see bubbles. Flip the pancake and continue cooking until both sides are lightly browned. Serve while still hot.

1 large banana, peeled and mashed (about ¾ cup)

2 large eggs

¼ cup unflavored carbonated mineral water

¼ teaspoon minced vanilla bean

1 scoop (10 grams) unflavored grass-fed collagen of choice (such as Vital Proteins)

Coconut or avocado oil, for frying

MAKES 2 SIDE SERVINGS
Prep time: 10 minutes
Cook time: 20 minutes

CARROT BACON

6 to 7 long, thick carrots

½ cup date syrup

Coconut oil spray

Himalayan sea salt

You now know that pork is off the table, owing to the reasons mentioned earlier in the book, and many turkey bacon and fake bacon options in the marketplace sadly contain gut irritants and additives. Well, that bacon flavor can still be enjoyed with this simple Carrot Bacon recipe! It's easily paired with eggs for protein, avocado for healthy fats (and deliciousness!), and of course your go-to Gut-Healing Frothy Coffee (page 216).

1   Preheat the oven to 400°F. Line a baking sheet with parchment paper.

2   Wash the carrots and slice them with a mandolin on the thickest setting, about ¼ inch. Then immerse each carrot slice, one at a time, in a small bowl filled with the date syrup to coat. Lay the carrot slices flat on the baking sheet.

3   Sprinkle the carrot slices with the salt, then bake for about 20 minutes, or until they begin to curl up and the edges begin to darken. Flip the slices and continue baking for another 10 minutes.

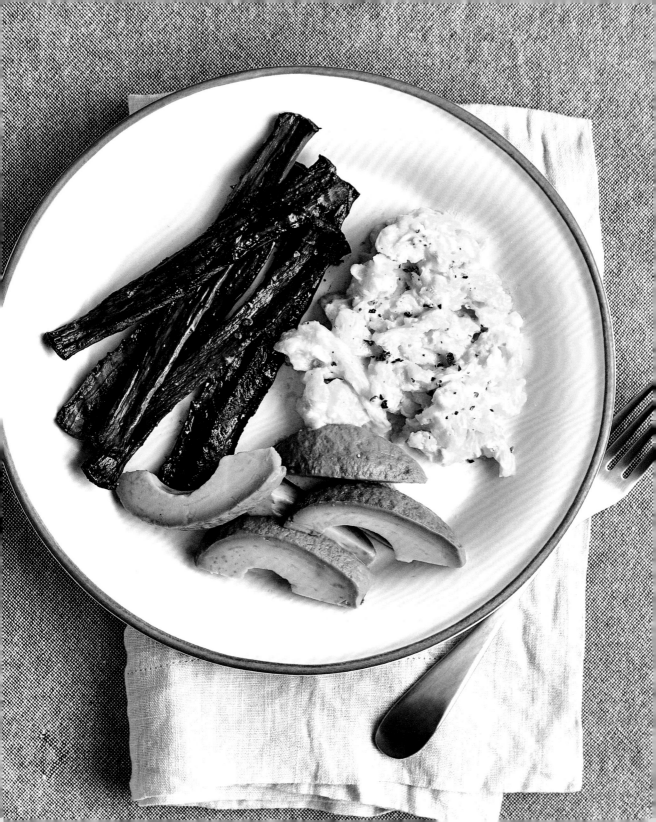

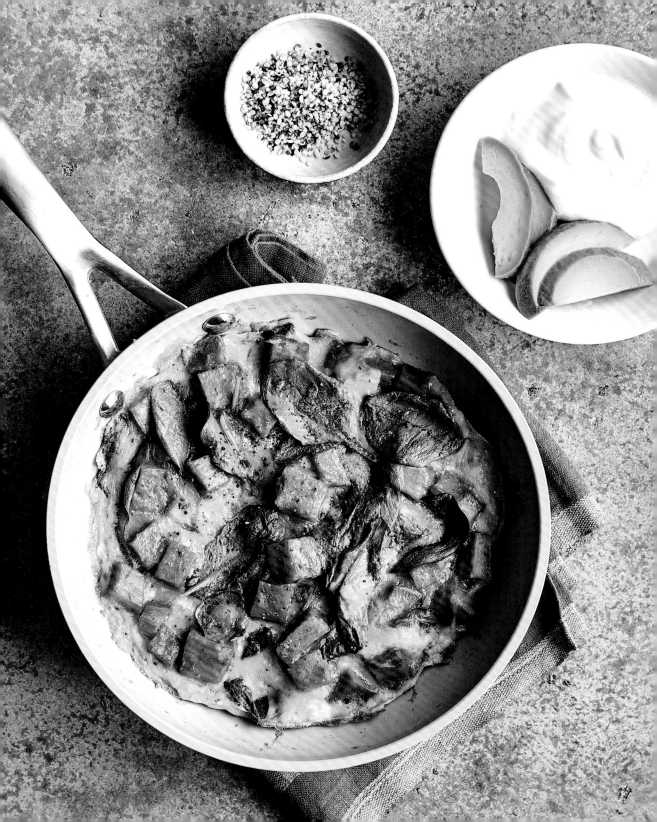

MAKES 1 SERVING
Prep time: 5 minutes
Cook time: 5 minutes

FIVE-MINUTE EGG HEMP HASH

I accidentally realized one day that you can make hash in 5 minutes; this happened when I didn't have any potatoes but I found prepped sweet potatoes in my freezer. I thought, *Hey, what the heck!* and I grabbed those pre-cut, pre-cooked chunks of sweet potato and tossed them in with the eggs and some fresh spinach. Five minutes later, the potatoes were thawed and cooked perfectly along with everything else! Sometimes having nothing on hand really can get your creative juices flowing.

1   Whisk the eggs in a bowl until frothy. Add the frozen sweet potato cubes and the spinach, and mix well.

2   Heat a medium skillet over medium heat and add the oil. Pour in the egg mixture and cook for 1 to 2 minutes, or until the eggs are fully cooked.

3   Transfer to a plate and garnish with the avocado, yogurt, and hemp seeds.

3 large eggs

½ cup frozen cooked sweet potato cubes (about 1 inch)

Handful of fresh spinach

1 to 2 tablespoons hempseed oil

½ avocado, peeled and seeded

¼ cup plain whole-milk cultured Greek yogurt

2 tablespoons hemp seeds of choice (such as Evo Hemp)

MAIN DISH RECIPES

These recipes are great for lunch or dinner—or even brunch! Enjoy!

MAKES 1 SERVING
Prep time: 10 minutes
Chill time: 1 hour

GUT-HEALING "PB&J"

The classic—with a twist! By now you know that peanut butter won't be used in this recipe. But SunButter is honestly the next best thing! It looks like peanut butter, and I may even go as far as saying that it tastes even better than peanut butter! (You can be the judge on that one.) As long as you have some basic sandwich bread sliced and ready to go, this is made in a flash (and eaten up just as quickly!).

2 slices Best Basic Sandwich Bread
(page 103)

Organic SunButter

Collagen Strawberry Jam
(recipe at left)

Spread the bread slices with the desired amount of SunButter, add the jam, and enjoy!

COLLAGEN STRAWBERRY JAM

MAKES ABOUT 1½ CUPS

1 cup fresh hulled or frozen sliced strawberries

½ cup filtered water

1 scoop (10 grams) unflavored grass-fed gelatin of choice
(such as Vital Proteins)

1   Place the strawberries in a small saucepan with water to cover over high heat until it comes to a boil. Add the gelatin and stir well.

2   Remove the pan from the heat and carefully pour the mixture into a blender. Secure the lid, and blend on high until the mixture is smooth. Transfer the jam to a glass jar. Cover and refrigerate at least 1 hour, until cool. While cooling, the jam will gel, firming up.

MAKES 1 SERVING
Prep time: 20 minutes
Cook time: 10 minutes

STUFFED SWEET POTATO TACO

Forget the tortillas in this recipe! Load up a sweet potato with all your favorite taco fillings, grab a fork (and napkin), and enjoy the best stuffed "taco" while sitting out on the porch in the fresh air. This is also great to prepare ahead of time by cooking extra sweet potatoes and storing them in the fridge. Since you are already preparing the fillings, why not make extra for the days to come?

1 medium sweet potato, scrubbed

4 ounces grass-fed ground beef

Seasonings: ground cumin, cayenne, paprika, chili powder, and/or salt (optional)

TOPPINGS

¼ cup Hemp Crema (recipe follows)

2 tablespoons minced fresh cilantro

Sliced olives

¼ large avocado, peeled, seeded, and sliced or chopped

Salt and pepper (optional)

Cauliflower "Cheese," "Cheddar" version (optional; page 106)

1   Fill a medium pot with water. Boil the sweet potato until tender, about 15 minutes. Cut in half lengthwise.

2   With clean hands, mix the spices (if using) into the ground beef, then place in a small pot with boiling water to cover, and poach for 6 to 8 minutes, until fully cooked. With a slotted spoon, remove the beef and place on top of the sweet potato halves. Garnish with the toppings.

HEMP CREMA

MAKES ABOUT 2 CUPS

1 cup hemp seeds (such as Evo Hemp)

1½ cups filtered water

½ tablespoon onion powder

½ teaspoon sea salt

Place all the ingredients in a blender and blend until smooth. Store in a glass jar in the refrigerator for up to 5 days.

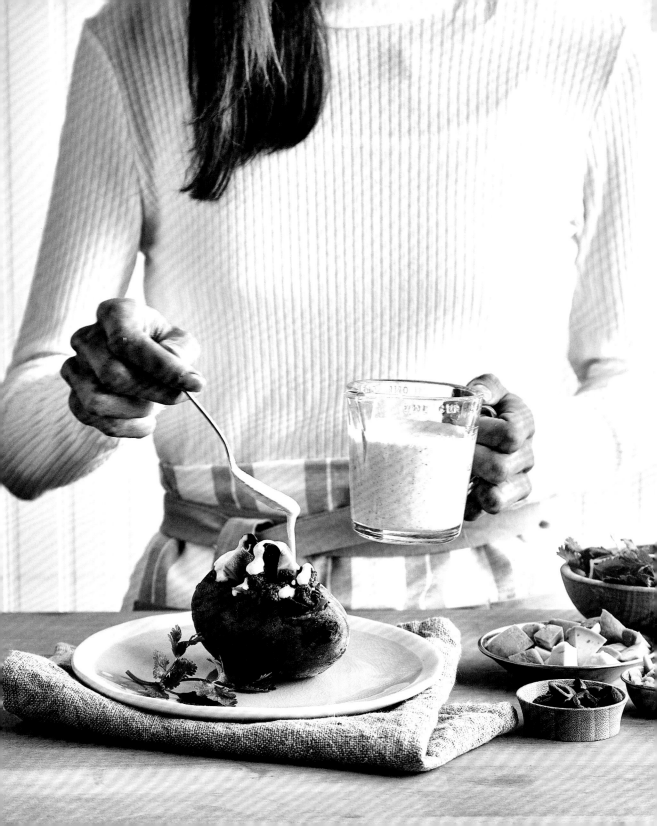

MAKES 1 SERVING
Prep time: 10 minutes
Cook time: 20 minutes

BAKED SWEET POTATO FRIES

with Sweet Yogurt Dipping Sauce

1 large sweet potato, scrubbed

Coconut or avocado oil spray

Sea salt

½ cup plain whole-milk cultured Greek yogurt

2 scoops (20 grams) unflavored grass-fed collagen of choice (such as Vital Proteins)

1 tablespoon raw honey

Who doesn't love a good sweet potato turned into crispy fries that are dipped into luscious Greek yogurt? Please, do yourself a favor and make this a regular. It's not only easy to make but also it's like dessert! And who doesn't want dessert as a main meal?

1   Preheat the oven to 400°F. Line a baking sheet with parchment paper.

2   Slice the sweet potato lengthwise into wedges. Lightly spray the wedges with oil and season with sea salt. Place the wedges on the baking sheet and bake for about 20 minutes, or until the edges are golden brown, turning halfway through.

3   Mix the yogurt, collagen, and honey in a bowl.

4   Serve the fries directly from the oven, along with the dipping sauce.

Corn is controversial in the IBS community; for many, the corn kernels can be difficult to digest. They can get caught in the digestive tract, causing a flare-up that may last for days. But if the corn is finely ground into flour and made into a tortilla, most people (including myself) have no problem digesting it! Just be sure there aren't any gums or additives in the ingredients when you are purchasing the tortillas (by now you're a pro at reading ingredients). Give these a try in a simple recipe that isn't just for Tuesdays. Tacos every day!

1 Preheat the oven to 350°F. Line a baking sheet with parchment paper.

2 Slice the tortillas into wedges with a pizza cutter, lightly spray the wedges with the oil, and place them on the baking sheet. Bake for 15 to 20 minutes, flipping halfway through, until the tortilla is crisp and edges are golden in color. Remove from the oven and allow to cool for at least 10 minutes (this allows them to crisp and harden like chips).

3 With clean hands, mix the spices (if using) into the ground meat, then place in a small pot, cover with boiling water, and poach for 6 to 8 minutes, until fully cooked. With a slotted spoon, remove the meat from the pot and set aside to cool.

4 Assemble the nachos by adding toppings of choice. Drizzle with the crema.

MAKES 2 SERVINGS
Prep time: 5 minutes
Cook time: 15 to 20 minutes

NACHO AVERAGE NACHOS

6 corn tortillas (from stone-ground masa meal)

Avocado or coconut oil spray

½ pound ground grass-fed beef or free-range turkey

Chili powder, ground cumin, and/or curry powder

TOPPINGS

Cauliflower "Cheese," "Cheddar" version (page 106)

Chopped avocado

Plain whole-milk cultured Greek yogurt

Sliced pitted olives

Minced fresh cilantro

Salsa of choice

Hemp Crema (page 154)

NO-COOK HEMP PASTA SALAD

1 8-ounce box lentil pasta

2 to 3 cups filtered water

½ can sliced pitted black olives

All-natural beef jerky or turkey jerky sticks, chopped (optional)

1 cup chopped ripe tomatoes (optional)

2 cups of Cauliflower "Cheese" (page 106)

1 large zucchini, chopped

2 to 3 tablespoons hempseed oil (such as Evo Hemp)

Hemp seeds, for garnish

Minced fresh basil leaves

Another time-saving trick I love is to soak the pasta. I've tried it with different varieties (chickpea and lentil), and find that the lentil-based pastas that contain no gums work best for this method. So, if you're short on time or just don't feel like standing over a hot stove, try this soaking method. It's also great for dorm-room meals or camping, if you don't have access to a stove. Try it!

1   Place the pasta in a large bowl and pour in enough filtered water to cover the pasta. Soak for about 45 minutes, or until the pasta is tender. Strain.

2   Add the olives, jerky sticks (if using), tomatoes (if using), Cauliflower "Cheese" cubes, and zucchini, and toss well.

3   Drizzle the hempseed oil and toss one more time. Garnish with some hemp seeds and fresh basil. Chill or serve immediately.

MAKES 4 SERVINGS
Prep time: 10 minutes
Cook time: 15 minutes

BETTER THAN MAC 'N' CHEESE

Did you grow up on mac 'n' cheese? Or perhaps this was a staple during your college years? Hey, no shame in the game for loving a good cheesy, carb-loaded dish! But needless to say, American cheese combined with glutinous pasta makes for a week in bed with stomach pains (at least for anyone with sensitive digestive issues). So, what's one to do when one craves this classic comfort dish? I've got you covered!

Cook the pasta according to the package directions. Strain and mix in a bowl with the sauce. Add the collagen (if using), and stir well.

1 8-ounce box chickpea pasta

1 recipe Nut-Free "Cheese" Sauce (recipe follows)

4 scoops (40 grams) unflavored collagen of choice (such as Vital Proteins, for added protein; optional)

NUT-FREE "CHEESE" SAUCE

MAKES ABOUT 2 CUPS

1 cup pumpkin puree (not pumpkin pie filling)

3 tablespoons organic SunButter

1 tablespoon yellow mustard

1 tablespoon onion salt

1 tablespoon apple cider vinegar

½ to 1 cup bone broth

Combine the ingredients in a blender with ½ cup of the broth until mixture is creamy. Add a bit more broth to make the sauce thinner, if desired. Can also be used as a dip.

BUTTER-NUT SQUASH AND APPLE SOUP

Butternut squash and apple were just meant to be together. Whether they're combined in a cold smoothie or a warm soup, this is a flavor combo everyone will enjoy! This soup can be served hot or cold.

1   In a saucepan set over medium heat, cook the squash, apples, and broth until the squash is tender, about 10 minutes. Carefully transfer the mix to a high-speed blender and add the SunButter. Blend well, until all the ingredients are creamy.

2   Pour the soup into bowls and serve with the biscuits.

4 cups peeled, seeded, and chopped butternut squash

2 large Honeycrisp apples, peeled, cored, and chopped

2 cups bone broth

2 tablespoons organic SunButter

Plain whole-milk cultured Greek yogurt (optional)

Basic Biscuits (page 105)

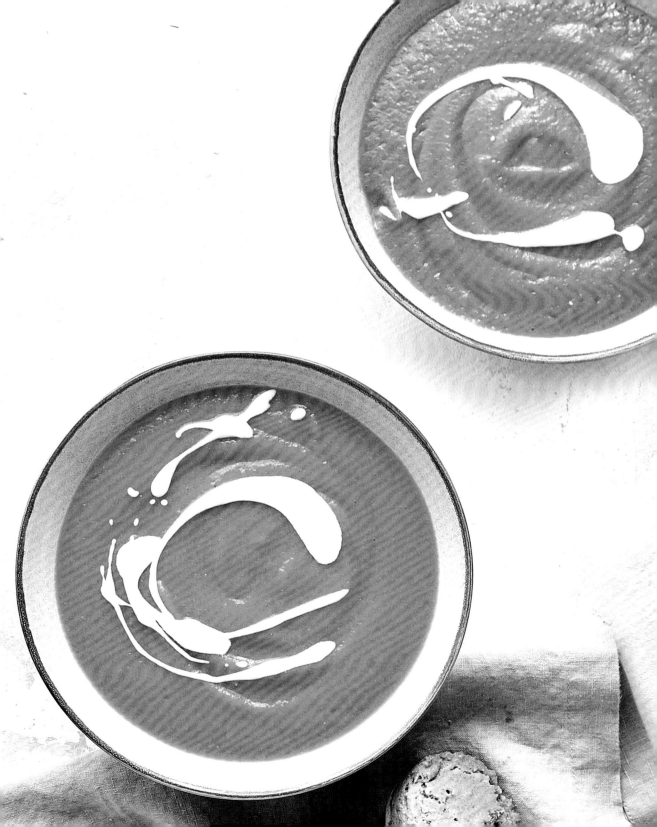

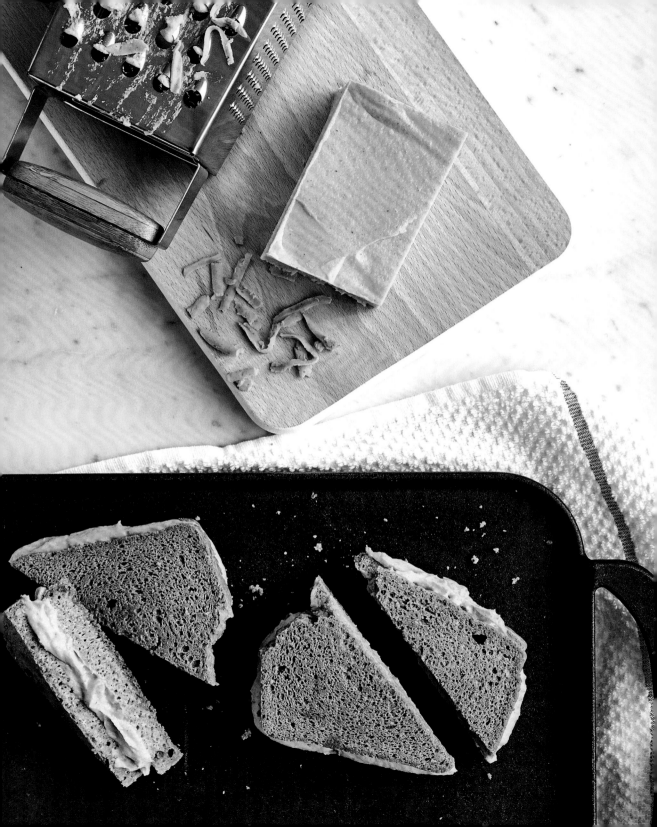

MAKES 1 SERVING
Prep time: 5 minutes
Cook time: 5 minutes

GRILLED (CAULI-FLOWER) "CHEESE" SAND-WICH

Here are two of my classic favorites combined into one! What could be better? We're taking gut health to the next level with this "cheesy" bite. Eat it alone or serve it with soup.

Heat a medium skillet with the oil over medium heat, then place a slice of bread in the pan and sprinkle the grated "cheese" evenly over it. Top with the other piece of bread. Grill until the edges are lightly browned, about 5 minutes, then flip to brown on the other side, another 5 minutes.

Avocado or coconut oil, for grilling

2 slices Best Basic Sandwich Bread (page 103)

½ cup grated Cauliflower "Cheese," "Cheddar" version (page 106)

ZESTY ZUC-CHINI TORTI-LLAS

2½ cups grated uncooked zucchini
(2 to 3 medium)

Seasonings of choice

2 scoops (20 grams) unflavored
grass-fed gelatin of choice
(such as Vital Proteins)

Move over cauliflower tortillas—there's a new veggie in town and his name is zucchini! I use grass-fed gelatin to make these tortillas 100 percent egg-free (for those needing that option). But even if you *can* eat eggs, this is just another fun and creative way to enjoy tacos and to keep your creative juices flowing in the kitchen!

1   Steam the grated zucchini for 30 to 60 seconds. Drain and transfer the wilted zucchini to a saucepan, then add the seasonings. Gradually sprinkle the gelatin into the saucepan while stirring over medium heat.

2   Line a large plate with parchment paper.

3   Transfer some of the zucchini to the plate and smash down in a circle. Layer with more parchment paper, then repeat with more of the zucchini, continuing to layer until all the zucchini is used. Wrap and refrigerate for at least 4 hours or overnight.

4   When ready, fill the tortillas as desired.

NOTE: The tortillas are best if filled with cold or room-temperature fillings, as any heat will soften the tortillas, owing to the gelatin.

MAKES 1 SERVING
Prep time: 10 minutes
Cook time: 5 minutes

TUNA MELT-YOUR-HEART SAND-WICH

There's a tuna melt on every diner's menu! It was always my go-to choice when dining out. It wasn't the best choice for overall health and optimal digestion, but with the simple changes I've made here, it's become one of the most gut-friendly melt-in-your-mouth sandwiches possible.

1   In a bowl, mix the tuna with the yogurt, salt and pepper (if using), and tomato (if using). Place the tuna mixture on one slice of bread, layer with the "cheese" slices, then top with the second slice of bread.

2   Place the sandwich in a toaster oven and toast until both sides of the bread are golden brown and the "cheese" is melted. (You can also grill the sandwich in a skillet on the stove top.)

1 5-ounce can tuna packed in water

¼ cup plain whole-milk cultured Greek yogurt

Salt and pepper (optional)

¼ cup diced ripe tomato (optional)

2 slices Best Basic Sandwich Bread (page 103)

2 slices Cauliflower "Cheese," "Cheddar" version (page 106)

MAKES 1 SERVING
Prep time: 5 minutes
Cook time: 5 minutes

LASAGNA SANDWICH

2 slices Best Basic Sandwich Bread
(page 103)

½ cup cooked grass-fed ground
beef or free-range turkey

¼ cup tomato sauce

Italian seasoning

⅓ cup cultured cottage cheese
(optional)

Several fresh basil leaves

Lasagna can be a lot of work. But this recipe is easy to assemble and quick to make! It has all the nutrient elements of lasagna, but with a healthy, easy-to-digest twist. And it's loaded with probiotics, protein, and, of course, flavor!

1   Toast the bread slices.

2   Mix the ground meat, tomato sauce, and seasoning in a bowl. Place one piece of toast on a plate. Spread the meat mix on the toast. Spread on the cottage cheese (if using), and add the basil leaves. Top with the second piece of toast and enjoy!

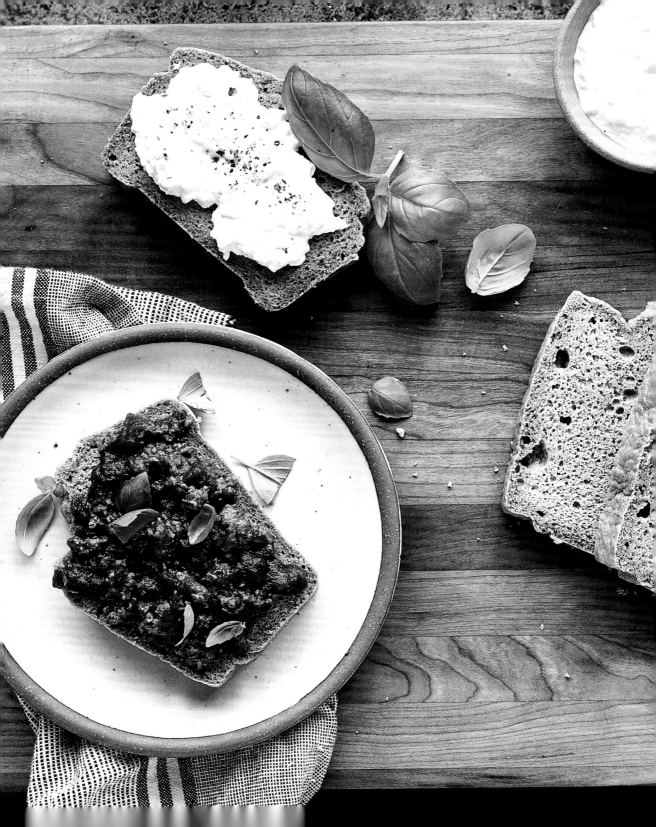

MAKES 2 SERVINGS
Prep time: 15 minutes
Cook time: 10 minutes

TOMATO-FREE BBQ SAUCE OVER GRILLED CHICKEN

2 cups chopped white onions
(about 2 medium)

½ cup filtered water

1½ cups fresh or
frozen pitted cherries

1 tablespoon apple cider vinegar

½ teaspoon ground cinnamon

¼ cup raisins

2 grilled 4-ounce chicken breasts

Your week just got better with this tomato-free sauce that you'll soon be putting on everything in addition to grilled chicken! Naturally sweetened, with no gums or thickeners (as so many store-bought sauces have), this BBQ sauce smothering a piece of free-range chicken will make your neighbors start knocking at your door. Hey, if they do, perhaps you can teach them all about gut health (by now you're a pro, right?). The sauce also works well with kebabs, burgers, or alongside fries. The sauce makes 1½ cups. Save any remaining sauce in a glass jar and refrigerate it; it is even better the next day.

1   In a large saucepan set over medium heat, simmer the onion in the water, allowing it to sweat, stirring occasionally, for about 10 minutes or until the onion is caramelized.

2   Add the cherries, vinegar, cinnamon, and raisins, and simmer for 10 minutes on low heat (the juice released by the cherries will begin to steep the raisins, softening the mixture).

3   Transfer the mixture to a high-speed blender and blend for a few seconds, until pureed. Set aside or chill in the refrigerator until ready to serve.

4   When ready to serve, add desired amount of sauce over the grilled chicken with your side of choice. Store any leftovers in refrigerator in airtight container up to 3 days.

"TLC" SAND-WICH

So many staples in this recipe! Honestly, as long as you have these prepped and ready to go, this turkey, lettuce, and cream cheese sandwich really will be TLC to your gut! You can even assemble it in the evening in preparation for lunch the next day. Then all you have to do is grab and go as you head out the door in the morning!

Spread the bread slices with the "cream cheese" and layer with the lunch meat. Add the lettuce. It's ready to enjoy!

2 slices Best Basic Sandwich Bread (page 103)

Homemade Cultured "Cream Cheese" (page 107)

2 to 4 slices Homemade Lunch Meat (page 109)

Lettuce

MAKES 1 TO 4 SERVINGS
Prep time: 15 minutes
Cook time: 25 minutes

Anti-Inflammatory
CRISPY FRIES 'N' DIP

If you're a crispy fry lover, then this is for you! Don't even get me started on the anti-inflammatory dip. And yes, this combo can be a meal! You've got your carbs from the potatoes (always opt for new white or golden potatoes, since they're easier to digest), your fats and protein from the hemp seeds and yogurt, your probiotics from the yogurt, and of course, those anti-inflammatory benefits from the hemp! I like to make a large batch of the dip, then depending on whether I want this as a meal or a snack, I air-fry the appropriate amount of potatoes.

CRISPY FRIES

2 to 5 new white or golden potatoes
Avocado or coconut oil spray

1   Wash and cut the potatoes into 1-inch-thick wedges.

2   Lightly spritz the potatoes with oil and place in an air fryer, leaving room between each potato for air to circulate.

3   Set the air fryer to 400°F for about 25 minutes, rotating halfway through.

ANTI-INFLAMMATORY DIP

Handful of fresh cilantro
½ cup hemp seeds (such as Evo Hemp)
Juice from ½ lemon
½ cup plain whole-milk cultured Greek yogurt
½ cup filtered water

Place all the ingredients in a blender and blend until smooth. Store any leftovers in the refrigerator for up to 2 days.

GRAIN-FREE SPANISH RICE

By now you know that I'm certainly not a rice hater (how are you enjoying the rice–yogurt combo?), but sometimes it's nice to just try something new. After all, you are more likely to stick with eating healthy if you never get bored! This dish is perfect accompanied with my Bean-Free "Refried Beans" (page 172).

1   Place the cauliflower rice in a large pot over medium heat and stir in the broth, Tabasco, tomato paste, cumin, and white pepper. Cook until the cauliflower is soft and tender, about 5 minutes.

2   Sprinkle the gelatin into the pot and stir until dissolved. The texture should get "sticky" as the mixture. If warmed again, the texture will loosen. When ready to serve, transfer to a bowl, add any optional ingredients, and garnish with a squeeze of fresh lime and cilantro.

1 16-ounce package
frozen cauliflower rice

½ cup bone broth

¼ cup Tabasco (optional)

3 tablespoons tomato paste

1 teaspoon ground cumin

1 teaspoon ground white pepper

1 scoop (10 grams) unflavored
grass-fed gelatin of choice
(such as Vital Proteins)

Juice of 1 lime

Minced fresh cilantro

OPTIONAL ADD-INS

Chopped onions

Pitted black olives

Chopped bell peppers

Cracked black peppercorns

BEAN-FREE "REFRIED BEANS"

1 cup delicata squash puree
(see Note)

1 16-ounce package
cooked ground beef

2 tablespoons olive oil

OPTIONAL ADD-INS

Onion powder

Garlic powder

Ground cumin

Ground white pepper

Tomato sauce

Plain whole-milk cultured Greek
yogurt or cultured sour cream

Sea salt

Beans are a food many cannot digest easily, and they can cause tons of gas. (I think we've all experienced that!) And sadly, people often remove beans from their diet because of these uncomfortable effects. If you miss down-to-earth, "home-cooked" Mexican refried beans, then this alternative will surely have you leaping for joy. It may seem intimidating at first, but trust me—once you try it, you'll be hooked!

1　Blend the squash, beef, and olive oil in a blender until smooth and creamy. (You may need to add 1 tablespoon water or so to facilitate blending, depending on how powerful your blender is.)

2　Taste the puree. If desired, stir in any of the add-ins. Transfer to a bowl and refrigerate to allow the "beans" to become firm.

3　When ready to serve, transfer the "beans" to a skillet and reheat.

NOTE: For the squash, roast about 2 cups chopped squash until soft and then puree in a blender without adding any liquid. Butternut squash will also work here.

MAKES 2 SERVINGS
Prep time: 10 minutes
Cook time: 15 minutes

CHEESE-BURGER SOUP AND CRISPY FRIES

Who knew a cheeseburger could become a soup? And be healthy at that! Yes, this combo is a little unusual, but thinking outside the box is something I've gotten used to doing. Dip these fries into your soup for the ultimate gut-healthy "burger" experience.

1   Brown the onion in a large skillet over medium heat until translucent, about 5 minutes. Add the remaining ingredients except the avocado. Adjust the seasonings to taste and simmer for 10 minutes.

2   When ready to serve, spoon the soup into a bowl, top with the avocado, dollop with a bit of ketchup, and serve with the fries.

1 medium white or yellow onion, chopped

1 medium butternut squash, roasted and flesh scooped out (about 4 cups puree)

1 tablespoon organic SunButter

2 garlic cloves

½ tablespoon yellow mustard

2 tablespoons tomato ketchup, plus additional for serving

½ teaspoon curry powder

1½ cups bone broth

10 ounces cooked ground beef or turkey

Slices of avocado

1 recipe Anti-Inflammatory Crispy Fries (page 170), made while soup is simmering

MAKES 2 SERVINGS
Prep time: 10 minutes
Cook time: 10 minutes

HEALTHY CHINESE "TAKE-OUT"

1 16-ounce bag
frozen mixed vegetables

1 cup frozen cooked shrimp

1 long carrot, peeled and then cut
into strips with a potato peeler

1 large (or 2 small) zucchini,
spiralized (or cut into strips
with a potato peeler)

1 tablespoon coconut aminos

1 tablespoon unsulfured
blackstrap molasses

Chinese on the cheap! Literally! Not only does this recipe give you all the tastiness of eating Chinese takeout but it's easily made right at home.

In a large skillet over medium heat, toss the vegetables, shrimp, carrot, and zucchini to mix well, then add the aminos and molasses. Cook until warmed through and coated with sauce. (You can add more sauce if desired; just add equal amounts of aminos and molasses.)

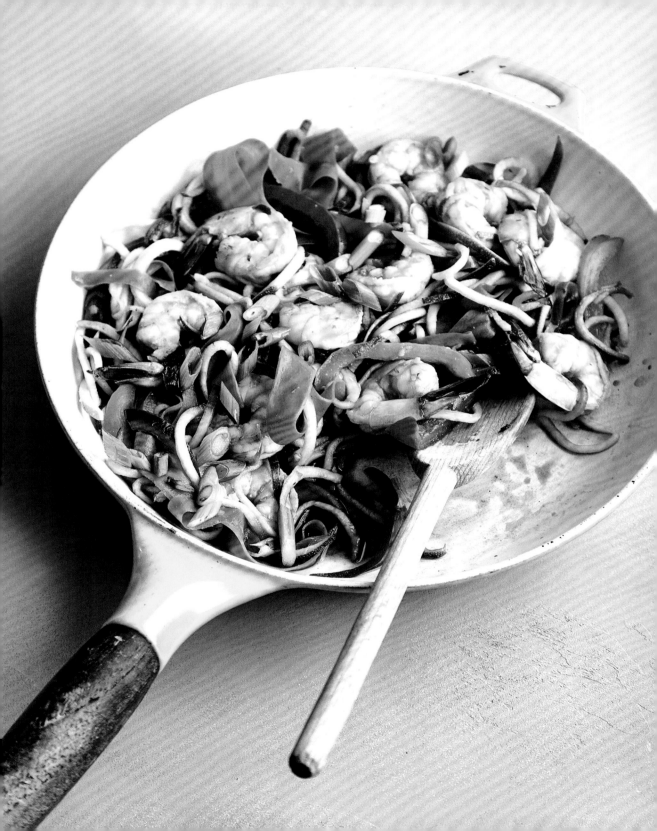

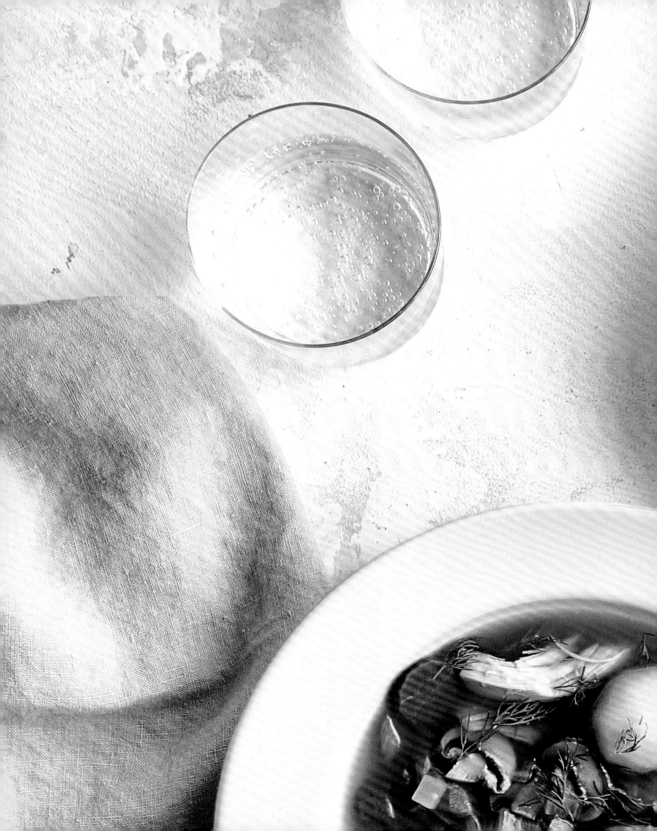

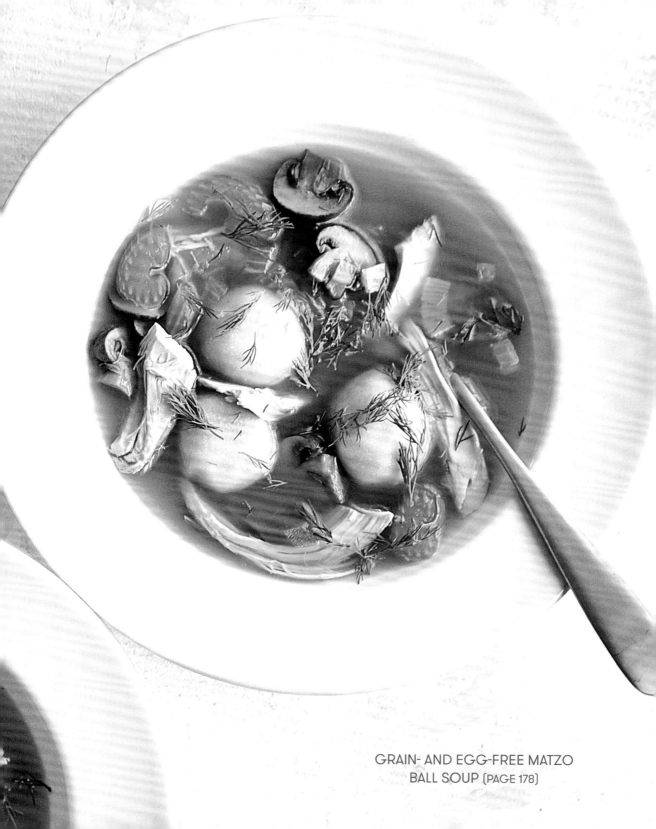

GRAIN- AND EGG-FREE MATZO
BALL SOUP (PAGE 178)

Grain- and Egg-Free

MATZO BALL SOUP

MATZO BALLS

½ cup cassava flour

2 teaspoons ground white pepper

1 teaspoon sea salt

1 tablespoon hempseed oil of choice (such as Evo Hemp)

6 tablespoons warm water

SOUP

4 cups bone broth, either chicken or beef

1 pound pre-cooked shredded chicken breast

2 cups cooked vegetables of choice (such as carrots, mushrooms, onions)

Ever had matzo ball soup? It's a traditional Jewish chicken soup with dumplings typically made from matzo meal (unleavened), eggs, and butter and often served during Passover. This version is a lot more gut-friendly and is also grain-, gluten-, dairy-, and egg-free!

1   Mix the cassava flour, white pepper, and salt in a large bowl, then add the hempseed oil and water, and mix until a dough forms.

2   Roll the dough into balls of 1 to 2 inches in diameter and drop into a large pot of boiling water. Allow the dumplings to cook for at least 10 minutes (time will vary depending on the size of balls), until they float to the surface.

3   In the meantime, bring the bone broth to a boil in a large pot over high heat; add the chicken and vegetables, reduce the heat, and simmer for 10 minutes.

4   If serving immediately, add the matzo balls to the soup. Alternatively, wrap and store them in the fridge for another day, to add to the hot soup.

MAKES 1 TO 2 SERVINGS
Prep time: 5 minutes
Cook time: 5 minutes

CHINESE FRIED "RICE"

You come home from work, look in the fridge, and find it's empty except for a carton of eggs; there are packages of cauliflower and frozen veggies in the freezer. Enter this quick and easy meal that is not only budget-friendly but also good for you. Perfect for any night of the week!

Coconut oil or avocado oil spray

2 cups frozen cauliflower rice

½ cup frozen chopped veggies

2 tablespoons coconut aminos

2 tablespoons unsulfured blackstrap molasses

2 to 4 large eggs

1   Coat a large skillet with the coconut oil spray and place over low heat. Add the cauliflower rice, veggies, coconut aminos, and molasses, and sauté until veggies are tender, about 3 to 5 minutes.

2   Scramble the eggs and then pour them onto the veggies in the skillet, and sauté 1 to 2 minutes, until the eggs are fully cooked. Serve at once.

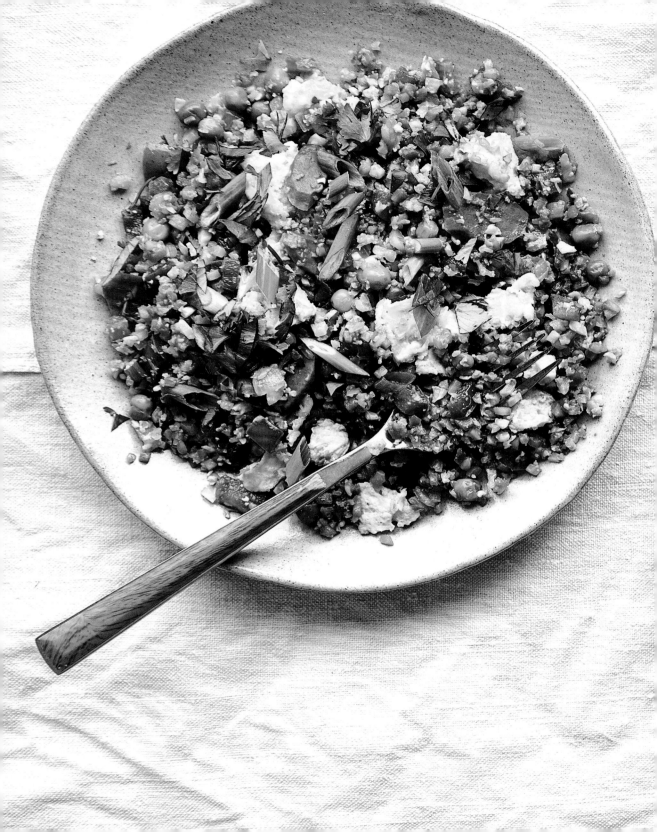

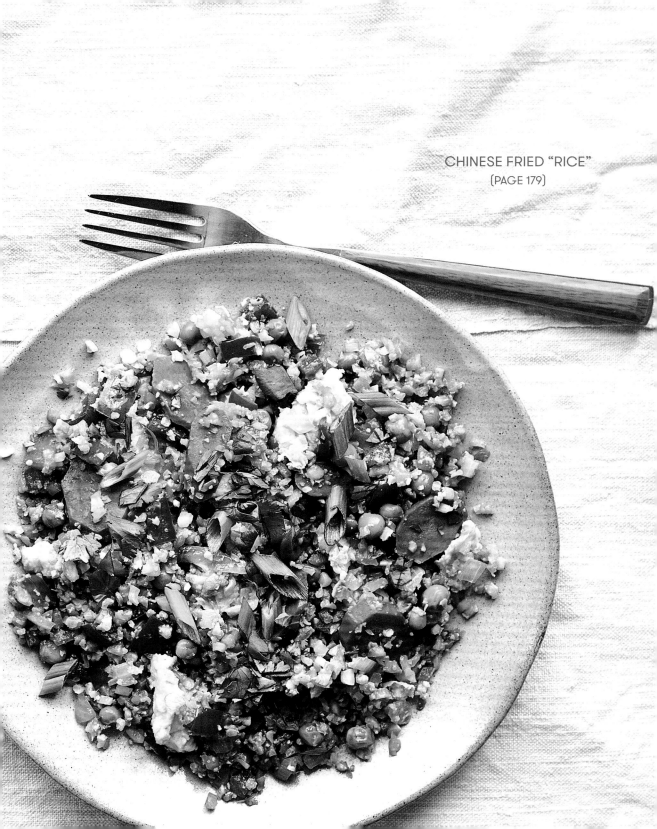

CHINESE FRIED "RICE"
(PAGE 179)

CHILLED AVOCADO-CUCUMBER MINT SOUP

2 large avocados

1 cup plain whole-milk cultured Greek yogurt

4 large cucumbers, peeled

¼ cup firmly packed fresh mint leaves

¼ cup firmly packed fresh cilantro

2 cups cold chicken bone broth

Juice of 1 small lime

Sea salt

Raw honey (optional)

Light, fresh, and gut-healing! This cold soup is perfect for those summer nights when you don't feel like cooking, or even turning on your stove, or putting in much effort. It's packed with protein, loaded with probiotics, and is super hydrating from the cucumbers. It's even great to make a double batch of this for your lunch the next day. You could also top the soup with cooked seafood of your choice (shrimp, crab, salmon, or tuna).

In a blender, combine all the ingredients except the honey until creamy. Adjust the seasoning to taste, and serve chilled with a drizzle of raw honey (trust me, it's amazing!).

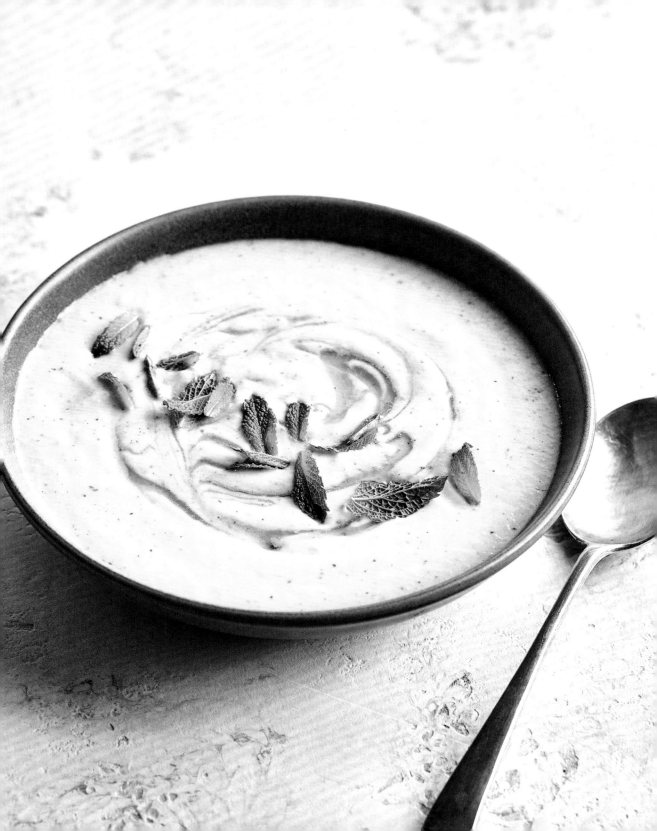

MAKES 4 TO 6 SERVINGS
Prep time: 10 minutes
Cook time: 30 minutes

TEXAS CHILI

with
Cauliflower "Cheese"

20 ounces ground free-range turkey

1 medium white onion, chopped

Avocado or coconut oil, for cooking

¼ teaspoon ground cumin

¼ teaspoon garlic powder

1 to 2 tablespoons chili powder

2 cups diced ripe tomatoes

1 16-ounce can tomato sauce

2 cups bone broth

2 16-ounce cans organic kidney beans (I like Trader Joe's)

Plain whole-milk cultured Greek yogurt

Grated Cauliflower "Cheese" (optional; page 106)

This dinner is one of those you'll crave after coming home from church on a Sunday afternoon. You know the routine. You all sit around the table, get out a board game, and enjoy a bowl of chili with family and friends! You'd better make extra, because everyone will want a bowl—you don't have to have digestive issues to enjoy this chili.

1 Place the turkey and onions in a deep pot along with a little oil, set over medium heat. Add the spices and continue to cook until the turkey is done, 8 to 10 minutes.

2 Add the tomatoes, tomato sauce, and broth. Stir well, then add the beans and simmer for about 20 minutes over low heat; the chili will thicken.

3 When ready to serve, scoop out into bowls and garnish with a spoonful of yogurt and a sprinkling of grated "cheese."

TEXAS CHILI "CHEESE" FRIES

Did you ever think you could eat chili "cheese" fries on a gut-healing diet? Well, with this healthy recipe you certainly can! My version uses air-fried potatoes for the ultimate comfort food that will fill you up, *not* out.

Place each serving of fries in a bowl and top with some chili.

1 recipe Texas Chili with Cauliflower "Cheese" (page 184)

1 recipe Crispy Fries (page 170)

MAKES 1 PIZZA, SERVING 2
Prep time: 10 minutes
Cook time: 20 minutes

CHICKEN PIZZA

1 12-ounce can
chicken meat (or tuna)

1 large egg

½ scoop (5 grams) unflavored
grass-fed gelatin of choice
(such as Vital Proteins)

1 teaspoon ground white pepper

TOPPING IDEAS

Cauliflower "Cheese," "Mozzarella"
version (page 106)

Slices of ripe tomato

Sliced pitted olives

Pineapple slices

Zucchini slices

This may be unusual and seem a little intimidating, but that's sometimes the case when you see a new recipe. I bet you thought that of some of the previous recipes in this book, but by now you're making them on a regular basis—no sweat! So this recipe is a piece of cake (I mean, slice of pie!). The protein is in the crust, so you can get creative with the toppings.

1   Preheat the oven to 400°F. Line a baking sheet with parchment paper.

2   Drain the chicken and place it in a blender or food processor along with the egg. Process until smooth. Add the gelatin and white pepper, and blend again until smooth.

3   Pour the puree onto the baking sheet and spread out with the back of a spoon to the desired shape and thickness (not too thick, but not too thin). Bake for 15 to 20 minutes, until the edges of the crust are crisp and light brown and the cheese has melted.

4   Top the crust with your desired toppings, then place back in the oven for a few minutes more if you want your toppings warmed and melted. Cut into slices and enjoy.

MAKES 4 SERVINGS
Prep time: 5 minutes
Cook time: 15 minutes

TACO PASTA

When two nationalities collide, there's a party in your mouth (and no party in your tummy, a win–win!). This is an easy, "throw-it-all-together" type of dish for when you need to feed a family quickly and simply (or just want to have extra for the days to come). In less than 30 minutes you'll have dinner cooked and on the table!

1   Cook the pasta in boiling water for 3 to 5 minutes, until al dente. Drain and set on a platter or plates.

2   In a large pot, combine the remaining ingredients except the cilantro, and stir over medium heat until it begins to boil. Reduce the heat and simmer for 5 minutes to blend the flavors.

3   Spoon the sauce over the pasta, stir a bit if desired, then garnish with the cilantro. Enjoy!

2 cups chickpea or lentil pasta

1½ cups shredded cooked chicken or ground meat

1½ cups tomato sauce

2 cups bone broth

2 tablespoons natural taco seasoning

1 large ripe tomato, diced

½ cup diced onion (optional)

¼ cup sliced pitted black olives

Fresh cilantro, to garnish

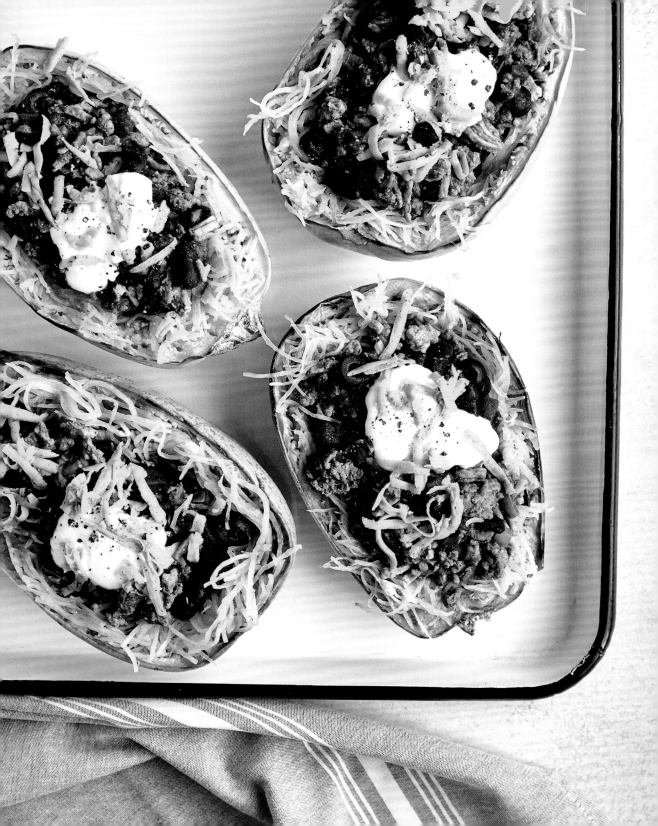

MAKES 4 SERVINGS
Prep time: 5 minutes
Cook time: 30 minutes

CHILI-STUFFED SPAGHETTI SQUASH

Ever had spaghetti squash? It's fun to eat, and there's no denying why it's named as it is. After it is cooked, you can comb out the flesh to get a dish of spaghetti-like strands. The squash has a high water content (great for digestion), and is also the perfect vessel for stuffing with just about anything!

1   Place the turkey and onion in a deep pot along with the oil and cook over medium heat for 5 minutes. Add the cumin and continue to cook until the turkey is cooked through, 8 to 10 minutes.

2   Add the tomatoes, olives, tomato sauce, and broth, and simmer for about 20 minutes over low heat, allowing the chili to thicken. Stir in the beans.

3   Loosen the squash halves by combing with a fork to form "pasta" strands. Fill each squash half with some of the chili. Transfer to plates, and garnish with a dollop of yogurt and a sprinkle of grated "cheese."

20 ounces ground free-range turkey

1 medium white onion, chopped

Drizzle of avocado or coconut oil

¼ teaspoon ground cumin

2 cups diced ripe tomatoes

½ cup sliced pitted black olives

1 16-ounce can tomato sauce

2 cups bone broth

2 16-ounce cans organic kidney beans

2 small spaghetti squash,
halved and roasted

Plain whole-milk cultured
Greek yogurt

Cauliflower "Cheese" (page 106)

MAKES: 4 SERVINGS
Prep time: 10 minutes
Cook time: 15 minutes

Grain-Free
BUTTER-NUT PASTA

This recipe is perfect for a family of four, and even more perfect to make just for yourself, with extras for the following days! Get creative by adding your favorite pasta flavorings (such as artichokes or olives), or keep it as is. You can even serve this with some toasted Best Basic Sandwich Bread slices (page 103). Feel free to add some grilled chicken for extra protein.

1 medium butternut squash

1 24-ounce jar "clean" pasta sauce, or your own

½ cup bone broth

2 to 3 cups shredded cooked chicken

½ cup chopped fresh mushrooms

1 large zucchini, cut into ¼-inch slices

Fresh basil, to garnish

1   Preheat the oven to 400°F. Line a baking sheet with parchment paper.

2   Peel the butternut squash with a potato peeler. Spiralize only the neck of the squash. Set the bottom part of the squash aside for another use.

3   Lay out the spiralized squash "noodles" on the baking sheet and bake for 10 to 15 minutes, or until noodles are tender.

4   Meanwhile, combine the pasta sauce, broth, chicken, mushrooms, and zucchini in a large saucepan placed over low heat and simmer until the veggies have softened and the chicken is heated through, about 10 minutes.

5   Transfer the baked "noodles" to a platter and top with the sauce. Garnish with fresh basil and serve at once.

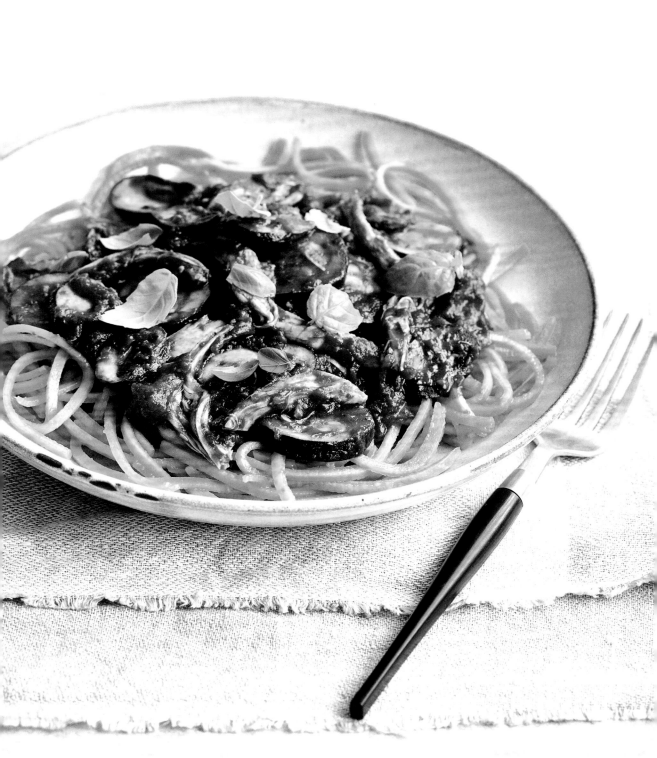

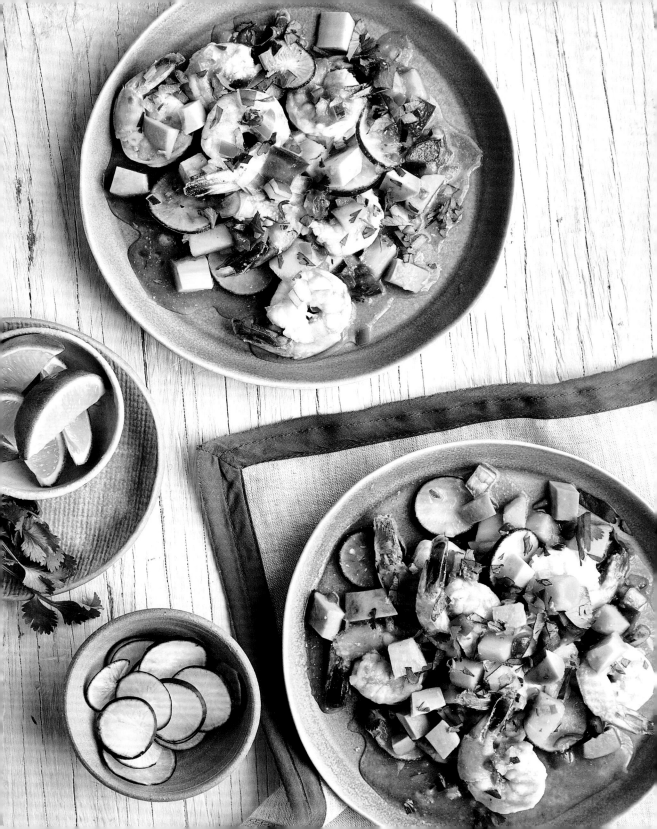

BONE BROTH SHRIMP "CEVICHE"

Ceviche is probably my favorite way to enjoy shrimp! As I retrained my taste buds, I learned to enjoy the natural flavors of various ingredients, and all the flavors in this ceviche really speak to me on a deep level! And I mean, who doesn't love a fun and creative way to enjoy bone broth on a hot summer night?

Combine all the ingredients except the cilantro in a large bowl. Chill well. When ready to serve, sprinkle with the cilantro.

1½ quarts filtered water

2 cups grilled or cooked shrimp

2 cups bone broth

2 tablespoons pink Himalayan salt

Juice from 2 limes

½ cup fresh tomato juice

3 to 4 radishes, thinly sliced (optional)

¾ cup chopped ripe mango

½ cup finely chopped onion

2 serrano chiles, seeded and finely chopped

¾ cup diced ripe tomatoes

1 large avocado, peeled, pitted, and chopped

Fresh cilantro, to taste

SNACK RECIPES

Forget snacking on the typical chips or junk food. These gut-healthy snacks will keep your energy up during busy days, as well as be a great go-to for parties and get-togethers.

PROTEIN FLUFF

This is my main, my go-to, my no-fail snack whenever I'm pressed for time, or need some extra protein, or am having tummy trouble, or just want a delicious chocolate snack! This fluff is it! It's full of probiotics and L-glutamine to help with gut repair and overall digestion. IBS flare-up or not, this fluff will be your best friend.

2 scoops (25 grams) chocolate protein powder of choice (such as my Probiotic Cacao Nuzest Protein Powder)

About ½ cup filtered water

In a glass, mix the protein powder with half the water, then gradually add more water until you get the right consistency of pudding or "fluff." Enjoy at once.

MAKES 2 SERVINGS
Prep time: 10 minutes
Cook time: 15 minutes

Anti-Inflammatory

AVOCADO VEGGIE PROTEIN DIP AND FRIES

⅔ cup frozen peas

½ cup frozen Brussels sprouts

1 small avocado, peeled, pitted, and sliced

¼ cup hemp seeds (such as Evo Hemp)

Juice of 1 lemon

Sea salt

Crispy Fries (page 170)

Of course, you have to have a classic here. Plain old taters crisped to perfection in an air fryer is something no one can turn down as a good, healthy snack. And paired with a dip designed to help with inflammation, there's really no excuse not to make these.

1 Boil about 1 quart of water, then pour over the frozen veggies in a bowl until they are submerged. Allow them to sit a few minutes, until thawed. (This is a way to steam them without making them mushy and they retain their bright vibrant green color.)

2 Drain the veggies, then combine with the avocado, hemp seeds, and lemon juice in a small blender and puree until smooth.

3 Taste, then add salt as desired and blend again. Serve as a dip with Crispy Fries.

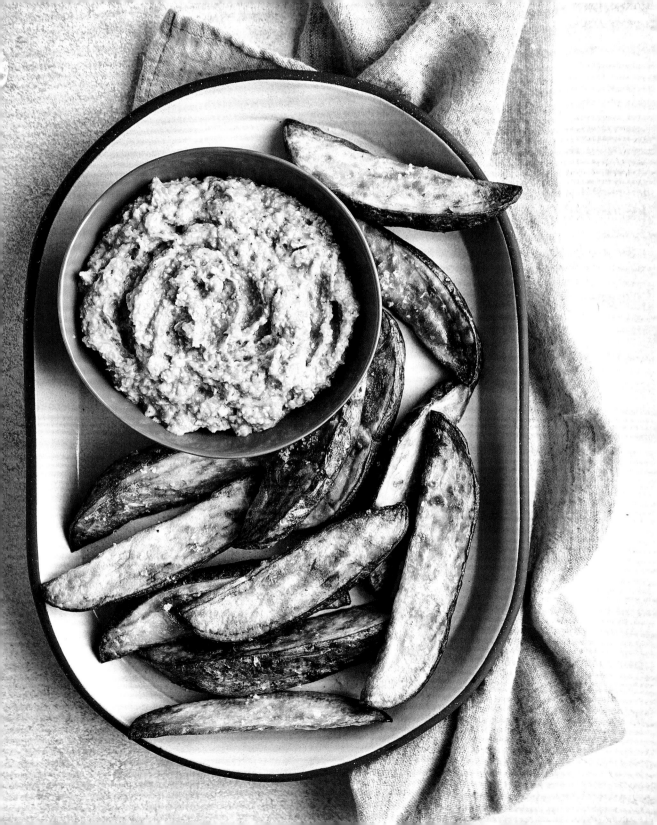

MAKES 2 SERVINGS
Prep time: 10 minutes
Cook time: 5 minutes

LOW-CARB CHOCOLATE GRAHAM CRACKERS

¼ cup unsweetened cocoa powder

2 scoops (25 grams) chocolate protein powder of choice (such as my Probiotic Cacao Nuzest Protein Powder)

½ teaspoon ground cinnamon

2 tablespoons coconut oil, melted

4 tablespoons filtered water

Who says crackers have to be savory? This chocolate version kind of reminds me of those tiny Teddy Grahams back in the day. I would beg my mom to buy them for me every time we grocery shopped, but she did so every once in a while, mostly for special occasions. Well, that craving stuck with me and that's why these chocolate crackers were created!

1   Preheat the oven to 350°F. Line a baking sheet with parchment paper.

2   Mix the cocoa powder, protein powder, and cinnamon in a large bowl, then add the coconut oil and water, and mix well.

3   With your hands, form the batter into one large ball. Roll out the ball with a rolling pin between two sheets of parchment paper. Cut into 2-inch squares with a pizza cutter. Lay the squares on the baking sheet.

4   Bake for 4 to 5 minutes, or until the crackers start to brown (watch carefully as they can burn quickly). Cool the crackers on a rack; during cooling, they will get crispy. Pack the crackers into a container, if there are any left, and store for up to 2 days at room temperature!

MAKES 2 SERVINGS
Prep time: 10 minutes
Cook time: 5 minutes

CINNAMON TOAST CRACKERS

Who doesn't love a sweet cinnamon cracker? These are a cross between cinnamon toast cereal and graham crackers.

1 Preheat the oven to 400°F. Line a baking sheet with parchment paper.

2 Combine the dry ingredients, then add the honey, coconut oil, and 1 tablespoon water. If the batter is crumbly, add 1 more tablespoon of water and mix well to get a firm dough.

3 Compress the dough into one large ball with your hands, then place on the baking sheet and cover with another sheet of parchment paper. Roll with a rolling pin until the dough is as thin as you can get it without breaking.

4 Remove the top paper and cut into evenly shaped 1-inch squares with a pizza cutter. Bake for 4 to 5 minutes, or until golden brown. (Watch carefully as they will turn/burn quickly!)

5 Let crackers cool on a rack for at least 10 minutes (this will make them crispier!). If desired, lightly spray the squares with coconut oil and dust with coconut sugar.

½ cup blanched almond meal

2 scoops (25 grams) pea protein of choice (such as my Probiotic Vanilla Nuzest Protein Powder)

1 teaspoon ground cinnamon

1 tablespoon raw honey or pure maple syrup

2 tablespoons coconut oil, melted

1 to 2 tablespoons filtered water

Coconut oil spray (optional)

Coconut sugar (optional)

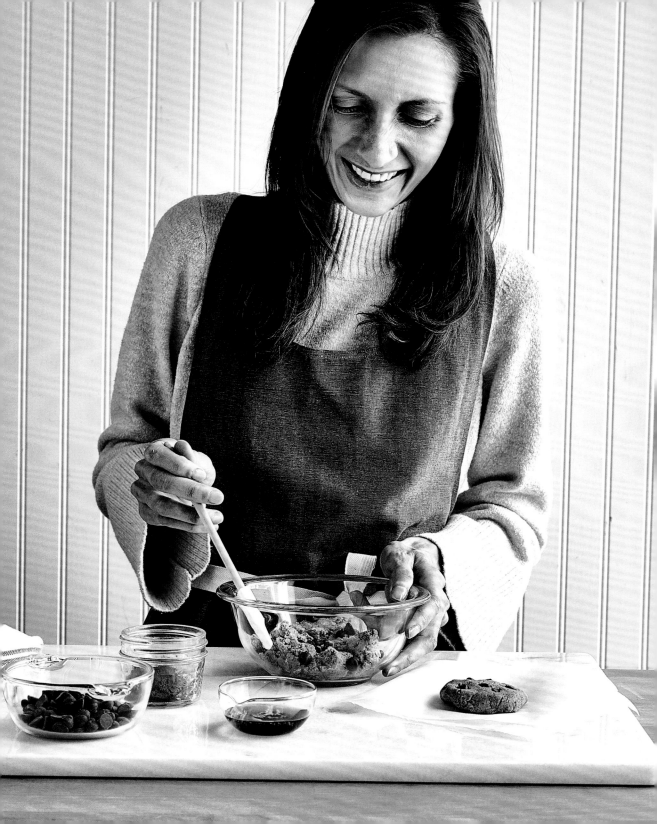

MAKES 1 COOKIE
Prep time: 5 minutes
Chill time: 5 minutes

60-SECOND PROTEIN COOKIE

Got 60 seconds? If you don't, I think you need to clear your schedule. Let's bypass the fact that this cookie is absolutely delicious and skip to the point that it's, once again, good for the gut! And unlike the packaged protein cookies you can always find at the gym, this is full of natural, anti-inflammatory ingredients.

1   Mix the protein powder, almond butter, cinnamon, coconut oil, and honey with 3 tablespoons of water. Add the chocolate chips and press the dough into one large ball with your hands. If dough is not sticking together, add 1 more tablespoon of water.

2   Form the dough into one large cookie (or several small cookie balls). Place in the freezer for 5 minutes to firm up. (I think it tastes even better chilled!)

2 scoops (25 grams) unflavored pea protein powder of choice (such as my Just Natural Nuzest Pea Protein Powder)

1 tablespoon smooth, "drippy" almond butter

½ teaspoon ground cinnamon

½ tablespoon coconut oil, melted

½ tablespoon raw honey

3 to 4 tablespoons filtered water

1 tablespoon unsweetened chocolate chips

MAKES 10 BALLS
Prep time: 10 minutes
Cook time: 5 minutes + 1 hour chill time

PROTEIN CAKE BATTER BALLS

2 scoops (25 grams) pea protein powder of choice (such as my Probiotic Vanilla Nuzest Protein Powder)

3 tablespoons coconut flour

½ cup filtered water

1 tablespoon coconut oil

2 tablespoons coconut butter (creamed coconut)

½ teaspoon vanilla extract

3 tablespoons coconut sugar (optional)

Where are my cake batter fans? And if you're not a fan, you may be converted after trying this easy recipe! You can double or even triple the batch for a "cake batter party" and invite your friends to join in the fun! Remember—food is always better enjoyed with loved ones. These balls are easy, fast, and can be personalized by adding extra "mix-ins" so you never get bored.

1 Mix the protein powder and coconut flour in a large bowl, then add the water and mix again to obtain a smooth mix.

2 Melt the coconut oil and coconut butter together in a small saucepan over low heat, then add to the bowl along with the vanilla and coconut sugar (if using). Stir until well incorporated and it becomes a thick crumble.

3 With your hands or a tablespoon, shape balls by compressing the batter until it sticks together. You should be able to form 10 balls that are about 1 inch in diameter. (If you prefer, you can incorporate pure, organic, chemical-free sprinkles throughout the dough or just on top.)

4 Refrigerate the balls at least 1 hour, until firm. Serve and enjoy!

BONE BROTH VITAMIN C ICE POPS

Bone broth isn't just for cold winter days! You really can do so much with it, including freezing it for a refreshing, gut-healing, nourishing ice pop everyone can enjoy. Feel free to add extra fruit or substitute a favorite fruit (I love incorporating blueberries into these ice pops). Get creative and mix it up!

1 Slice the desired amount of kumquats and place them into your ice pop molds.

2 Mix the remaining ingredients, then pour into the molds and freeze for 1 hour or until completely frozen.

Kumquats, as needed

2 cups chicken bone broth

¼ cup orange juice

Juice of ½ lemon

CHICKEN CHIPS

2 cooked boneless and skinless chicken breasts

¾ cup warm water

2 scoops (20 grams) unflavored grass-fed gelatin of choice (such as Vital Proteins)

¼ cup cassava flour

2 teaspoons onion salt

Chicken—in chip form! These will literally blow your mind! Who ever thought you could eat chicken as crispy chips? They are perfect for those munchie cravings! Packed with protein and gut-healing benefits from the gelatin, they're also grain-, gluten-, and egg-free. You can dip these Paleo chicken chips into everything!

1   Preheat the oven to 350°F. Line a baking sheet with parchment paper.

2   Puree the chicken and water together in a blender until smooth; add the gelatin and blend again.

3   Add the cassava flour and onion salt, and puree one more time.

4   Drop small rounds of puree on the baking sheet and flatten with the back of a spoon (the thinner the better!). Bake for 20 to 25 minutes, or until they are crisp; the baking time will depend on how thin your chips are. Store any leftovers in an airtight container at room temperature for up to 2 days.

PALEO SPINACH DIP
(PAGE 206)

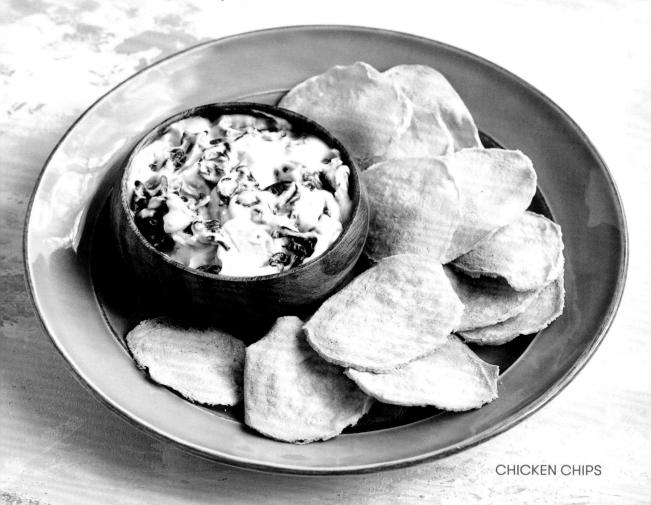

CHICKEN CHIPS

PALEO SPINACH DIP

1 medium head of cauliflower

2 scoops (20 grams) unflavored grass-fed collagen of choice (such as Vital Proteins)

2 to 3 tablespoons Paleo, vegan, or Whole30-approved mayo of choice

2 garlic cloves (optional)

1 to 2 teaspoons ground white pepper (optional)

Sea salt

½ cup water chestnuts

½ cup frozen artichoke hearts, thawed

1 16-ounce package frozen spinach, thawed and drained

Here's a dairy-free dip we can all gather around to enjoy munchies! I always make extra food and bring it to parties so I know I'll at least be able to share what I bring and won't feel "out of place" by not being able to eat at the gathering. This recipe is perfect for such occasions and can be enjoyed by everyone!

1   Steam the cauliflower until tender, then puree in a blender (do not add any water) until creamy.

2   Add the collagen, mayo, garlic (if using), and white pepper and blend again. Season with salt.

3   Cut the chestnuts and artichokes into smaller pieces, then fold into the cauliflower dip.

4   Add the spinach to your cauliflower dip, stir to blend, and chill before serving.

When I was a kid, my dad would always order cheesecake, since it was his favorite dessert. And he always shared it with me. As I got older, I realized how overly rich cheesecake is and how it doesn't sit well with me. Thankfully I don't have to give it up (and neither do you!) with this recipe. These truffles aren't overly sweet, nor do they make you want to take a nap after eating three of them. They're packed with nutrients, protein, and probiotics, and still satisfy that cheesecake craving. My dad would approve!

Mix all the ingredients well in a bowl until a firm dough forms. Scoop out and shape into balls about 1 inch in diameter. Enjoy at once or store any leftovers in the refrigerator.

FIVE-MINUTE "CHEESE CAKE" COOKIE DOUGH TRUFFLES

½ cup (37 grams) pea protein powder of choice (such as my Probiotic Vanilla Nuzest Protein Powder)

1 cup plain whole-milk cultured Greek yogurt

3 tablespoons organic SunButter

Unsweetened chocolate chips, as needed

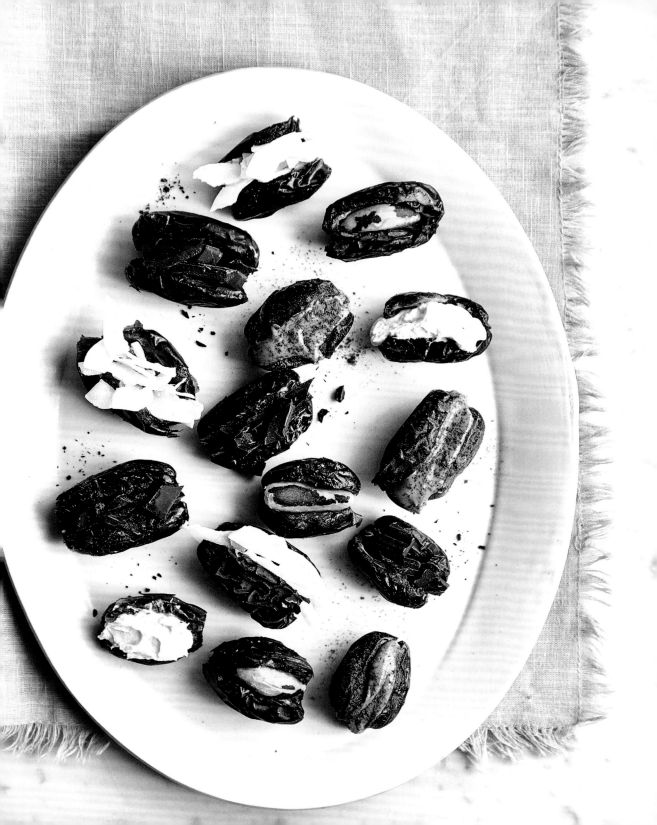

STUFFED DATES

Dates are nature's ultimate candy. Yes, dates are high in sugar, but does that mean you can never have them? Of course not! Remember, everything in moderation. I suggest eating just one date as a small, simple treat. One is enough to feed your brain, body, and soul.

Open each date and fill with the desired option. Enjoy!

8 large Medjool dates, pitted

FILLING OPTIONS

Organic SunButter and ground cinnamon

Whole Brazil nut

Pistachio butter

Homemade Cultured "Cream Cheese" (page 107)

Coconut shavings

Dark chocolate

Easy-Peasy

PROTEIN COOKIE DOUGH BITES

¼ cup creamy nut or seed butter of choice (SunButter, cashew, or almond)

3 scoops (37.5 grams) pea protein powder of choice (such as my Probiotic Vanilla Nuzest Protein Powder)

½ teaspoon ground cinnamon

½ cup filtered water

Unsweetened chocolate chips, as needed (optional)

These cookie dough bites will be gone in just as much time as it takes to make them! The recipe is one of my staples. They're the perfect little pick-me-up in the afternoon or evening, or even a great addition to a smoothie. This recipe can even be made nut-free for any nut allergens by using SunButter (or if you just want to mix it up in general). Simple, quick, and—dare I say—addicting!

Mix all the ingredients in a bowl and form into 9 equal balls about 1 inch in diameter. Store in the refrigerator for up to 4 days or freeze up to 3 weeks.

DRINK RECIPES

Drinks are sometimes overlooked in cookbooks, but they're a great way to get some gut-healing foods into your diet.

CREAMY MORNING MATCHA

2 cups warm water

1 tablespoon collagen matcha powder of choice (such as Vital Proteins)

1 teaspoon grass-fed ghee (clarified butter)

½ scoop (5 grams) unflavored grass-fed gelatin of choice (such as Vital Proteins)

If you want to switch up your coffee routine, what better way than to do it with a creamy cup of matcha? Just be sure the matcha is 100 percent pure (one ingredient, no fillers, flavorings, or sugars) and greet the morning with a boost of green tea antioxidants!

Combine all the ingredients in a high-speed blender and blend for 30 seconds, until smooth. Pour into a large cup and enjoy!

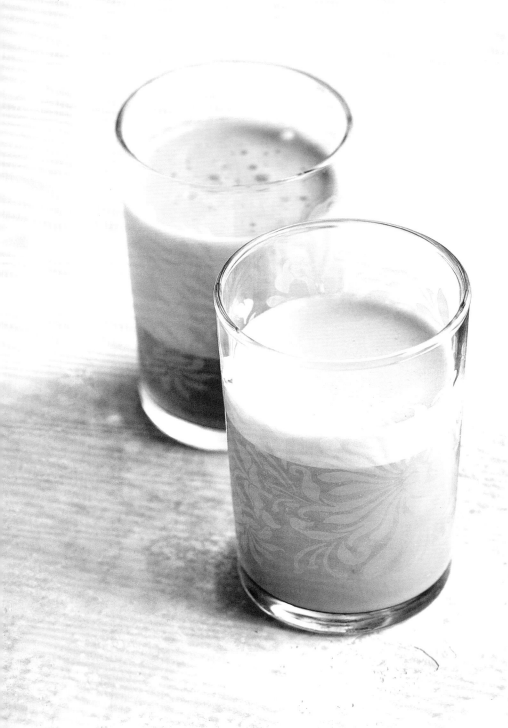

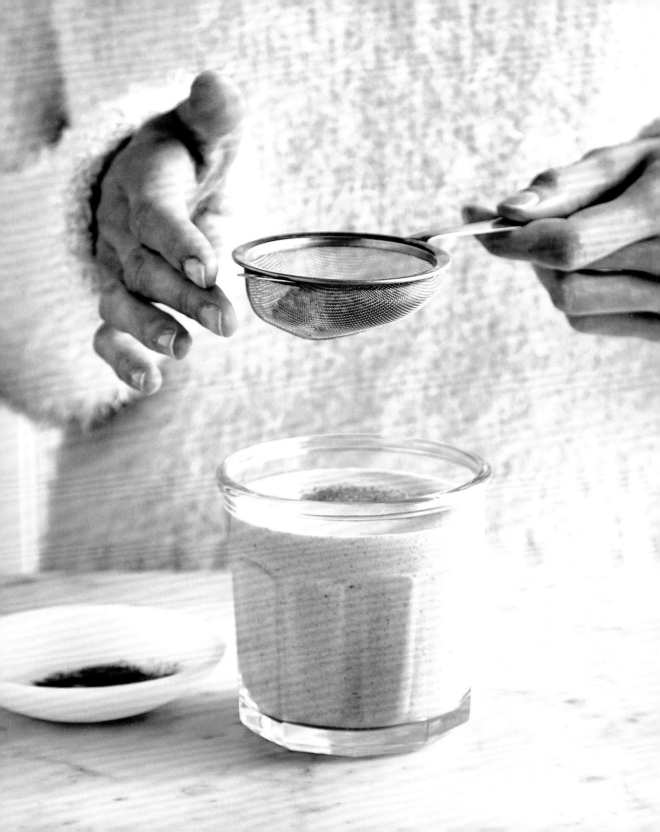

HOLIDAY OAT NOG

I love eggnog, but the raw eggs, processed sugar, and gums (yes, even the "traditional, clean" versions of many brands contain gums) just aren't worth it for me to indulge in a cup during the holidays. But not to worry! Try this dairy-free, egg-free, sprouted oat nog next time you get that craving. You may not be able to stop after just one glass of this creamy, thick drink!

2 cups old-fashioned rolled oats

4 Medjool dates, pitted

¼ teaspoon grated nutmeg

¼ teaspoon ground cinnamon

Pinch of sea salt

Juice from ½ lemon

3 cups water, plus more if needed

1   Combine the rest of the ingredients with the 3 cups water and store in the fridge overnight.

2   The next day, add the mixture to a blender and blend until creamy. At this point, taste the puree. If needed, adjust the seasonings to taste. Depending on preference, add more water and blend again to thin out or leave as is for a thicker consistency. Store in the refrigerator for up to 3 days.

GUT-HEALING FROTHY COFFEE

2 cups brewed coffee

1 teaspoon grass-fed ghee
(clarified butter)

1 scoop (10 grams) unflavored
grass-fed gelatin of choice
(such as Vital Proteins)

I admit it—I love coffee! But sadly, it doesn't love me, *except when I make it like this!* Time and time again I've received messages from people saying this is the only way they can drink coffee without upsetting their stomachs. There's actually a science behind this combination, though. Drinking this blended coffee recipe each morning helps your body burn fat all day, and can help you trim down. It also helps me stay regular.

Combine all the ingredients in a high-speed blender and blend for 30 seconds, until smooth and frothy. Pour into a large cup and enjoy!

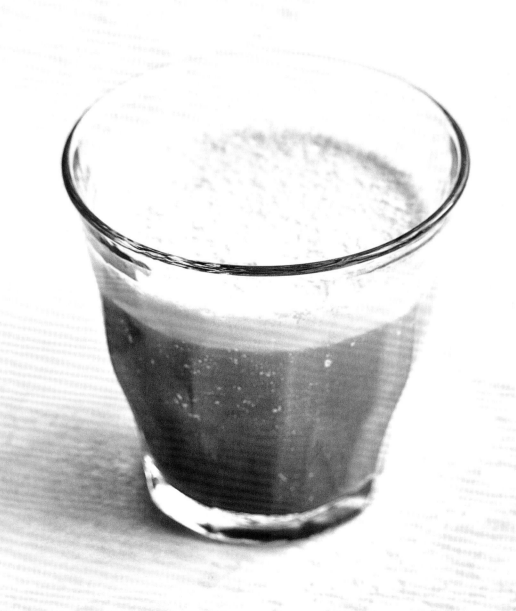

MAKES 2 TO 3 QUARTS
Prep time: 15 minutes
Cook time: 3 to 4 hours

HOMEMADE CHICKEN BONE BROTH

3 pounds chicken bones and feet (the more connective tissue on the bones, the better; look for knuckles, backs, necks, etc.)

3 cups chopped vegetables of choice (such as carrots, celery, leeks) (optional)

2 bay leaves

2 teaspoons sea salt

Filtered water

Nothing can be more comforting than homemade chicken bone broth. This recipe can actually be therapeutic for the mind. Listen to something calming while you chop the veggies, then "veg out" while the simmering takes place and fills your home with an aroma that will make your mouth water. There's no speeding up this process, as cooking it slowly is key, but the result is well worth it!

1   Place the bones, vegetables (if using), bay leaves, and salt in a large stockpot and pour in the filtered water until the contents are submerged.

2   Bring to a boil, then reduce the heat to low and simmer for 3 to 4 hours with the lid on, leaving a slight opening for steam to escape.

3   Allow to cool completely, then strain through a strainer. Pour the broth into glass jars and store in the refrigerator overnight.

4   Once chilled, the broth should be jiggly and a layer of fat should form on top. Skim the fat and reserve for other cooking uses or discard. Use the bone broth for drinking.

MILK IN 30 SECONDS!

This 30-second "milk" is not only easy but will also save you from spending tons of money, as well as conserving milk bottles and cartons. You'll never wake up and think "Yikes! I'm out of milk!" ever again (unless you're out of nut or seed butter—but if you're like me, you've always got a good stash on hand).

Place all the ingredients in a high-speed blender and blend for 30 seconds or until smooth. Pour into a glass jar and store in the refrigerator for up to 5 days. No straining required!

2 tablespoons of your favorite nut or seed butter (cashew, almond, SunButter, etc.)

2 cups filtered water

1 Medjool date, pitted (optional)

½ tablespoon sea salt (optional)

BONE BROTH LEMON- ADE

1½ cups bone broth

Juice from ½ lemon

½ tablespoon coconut sugar

3 to 4 ice cubes

Bone broth is great all year around, agreed? There's no excuse not to get in the gut-healing goodness during the summer months, when you have this recipe to keep you healthy, hydrated, and happy! You can make batches for those summer BBQs, picnics, and that week your air conditioner decides to give out (we've all been there).

Combine all the ingredients in a glass and enjoy!

One-Ingredient

RAW COCO- NUT MILK

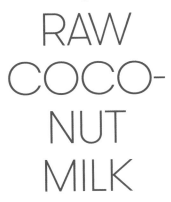

Say hello to the best coconut milk you will ever taste! It doesn't get much fresher than this. And with just one ingredient (as nature intended), it will spoil you for all the other coconut milks on the market (and keep your pocketbook happy, too!).

2 fresh young coconuts

4 cups filtered water (can include coconut water)

1 Carefully open the coconuts by using the dull edge of a knife to pierce the coconut until it breaks apart—nine times out of ten it will open in perfect halves. (Many grocery stores sell coconuts already halved.) Reserve the coconut water.

2 Scrape out the coconut meat and place in a blender with ½ cup water and/or coconut water and blend until smooth and creamy. Add the remaining 3½ cups of water and continue blending until smooth. Pour into a large glass jar and store in the refrigerator for up to 5 days.

CAFFEINE-FREE CREAMY HOT "COCOA"

2 cups hot water

½ tablespoon organic SunButter

2 teaspoons coconut sugar (optional)

1 tablespoon carob powder

1 scoop (10 grams) unflavored grass-fed gelatin of choice (such as Vital Proteins)

When you want a little something at night, but also want to get in those eight hours of sleep, enter this creamy cup of what may look like hot cocoa, but in fact is not! Can you tell the difference?

Combine all the ingredients in a high-speed blender and blend for 30 seconds, until smooth. Pour into a large cup and enjoy!

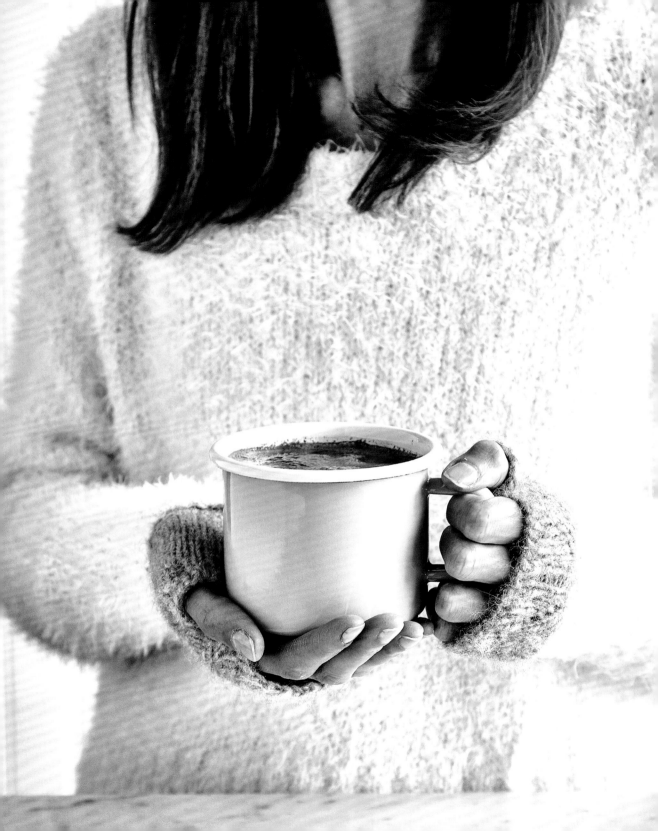

SPICY BONE BROTH HOT CHOCO- LATE

Cuddle up by the fireplace (or heater), light some candles, and get romantic with your cup of hot cocoa! I mean, what's life without a little spice in your chocolate love life?

Combine all the ingredients in a high-speed blender and blend for 30 seconds, until smooth. Pour into a large cup and enjoy!

2 cups bone broth

1 teaspoon coconut oil

1 teaspoon coconut butter (creamed coconut)

Dash of ground cinnamon

Dash of cayenne

2 teaspoons coconut sugar (optional)

2 tablespoons unsweetened cocoa powder

1 scoop (10 grams) unflavored grass-fed gelatin of choice (such as Vital Proteins)

DESSERT RECIPES

Yes, you can have dessert—even if you have IBS, and even if you're counting calories or watching your weight. My recipes are delicious, nutritious, and, best of all, they let you "indulge" with absolutely no guilt!

CARB-FREE CRUMB COOKIES

2 scoops (20 grams) unflavored grass-fed gelatin of choice (such as Vital Proteins)

1 scoop (12.5 grams) pea protein powder of choice (such as my Probiotic Vanilla Nuzest Protein Powder)

½ cup "drippy" almond butter

3 tablespoons hot water

Unsweetened chocolate chips or pieces to top, as desired

For when you've outdone it on the carbs for the day, or are on a candida diet, or just want a really good cookie, these will hit the spot! I call them "crumb cookies" because they tend to be a bit crumbly (not chewy, not hard, not crispy—almost like a biscuit!). I've made them so many times I know this recipe by heart (and you will too!).

1   Preheat the oven to 350°F. Line a baking sheet with parchment paper.

2   In a bowl, mix the gelatin with the protein powder; add the almond butter and hot water, and mix well. The dough should be thick, like Play-Doh.

3   Form the dough into 6 balls about 2 inches in diameter. Place on the baking sheet and press down to flatten them, if desired, or leave them round and plump. Bake for 10 to 15 minutes, or until their edges begin to brown.

4   Immediately after removing the cookies from the oven, top with some unsweetened chocolate chips or pieces. Allow to cool in the fridge (they also taste amazing frozen!) before eating.

MAKES 1 SMALL LOAF CAKE
Prep time: 10 minutes
Cook time: 30 to 35 minutes

ONE-BOWL CHOCOLATE COLLAGEN POUND CAKE

This recipe is a staple, and has been for years in my house. No sugar, no flour, no yeast, no gluten, and no unnecessary ingredients needed to create this decadent, rich chocolate pound cake everyone will love. You may want to double the batch and make two loaves because it will go fast!

1   Preheat the oven to 350°F. Grease an 8½ x 4½-inch loaf pan or line with parchment paper.

2   With an electric or stand mixer, beat the eggs and baking soda until foamy and doubled in volume, about 4 minutes. Add the cocoa powder, collagen, and almond butter, and continue mixing for 2 minutes, until the batter is smooth and creamy.

3   With a spoon, stir in the desired amount of chocolate chips (if using) and pour the batter into the loaf pan. Bake for 30 to 35 minutes, or until a toothpick inserted in the center comes out clean.

4   Let the loaf cool in the pan, then invert onto a rack to cool completely. Slice when cool and store in the refrigerator for up to 5 days or freeze for up to 2 months.

4 large eggs

1 teaspoon baking soda

½ cup unsweetened cocoa powder

2 scoops (20 grams) unflavored grass-fed collagen of choice (such as Vital Proteins)

1 cup creamy almond butter

Unsweetened chocolate chips, as needed (optional)

MAKES 1 SMALL LOAF CAKE
Prep time: 15 minutes
Cook time: 35 minutes

PALEO CARROT CAKE

Carrot cake can be intimidating to make since it does call for quite a lot of ingredients. But most of them are spices to get the flavor just right, and ingredients like raisins and coconut shreds are always optional if you're not a fan. I'm a *huge* fan of it all, and this loaf will surely get even the non-carrot-cake lovers' approval!

1 teaspoon baking soda

1 tablespoon apple cider vinegar

4 large eggs

½ cup "drippy" almond butter

½ cup cassava flour

1 cup grated raw carrots

1 teaspoon ground cinnamon

½ teaspoon grated nutmeg

½ cup finely shredded unsweetened coconut

⅓ cup small pineapple chunks

⅓ cup raisins, soaked in hot water for 15 minutes and drained

1 Preheat the oven to 350°F. Grease an 8½ x 4½-inch loaf pan or line with parchment paper.

2 Place the baking soda and vinegar in a large mixing bowl and let sit for a few minutes to fizz. Add the eggs and beat with an electric or stand mixer until foamy and doubled in volume.

3 Add the almond butter, cassava flour, grated carrots, cinnamon, nutmeg, and coconut, and continue to beat until well mixed.

4 Fold in the pineapple and raisins and then pour the batter into the loaf pan. Bake for about 35 minutes, or until a toothpick inserted in the center comes out clean.

5 Let cool in the pan and then invert onto a rack. Let cool completely before slicing. Store in the refrigerator for up to 2 days or freeze for up to 2 weeks.

CAULI-FLOWER RAISIN RICE PUDDING

If you can make "rice" from cauliflower, why not rice pudding from cauliflower rice? The juicy raisins plump up in this and add just the right amount of natural sweetness to each bite. Don't knock it 'til you try it! The amounts here are all suggestions. You can adjust the sweetness, cinnamon, and salt to taste and of course add more raisins if you're a raisin lover!

1   In a large pot, place the cauliflower rice and pour in enough water to cover, cooking until it is soft, about 3 minutes.

2   Soak the raisins (if using) in hot water to plump them.

3   Drain the cauliflower rice and add the honey (if using) to the pot, mixing until melted.

4   Add the yogurt, cinnamon, and sea salt, and stir well.

5   If adding raisins, drain them and add to the cauliflower mixture. Serve the pudding warm or chilled!

3 cups frozen cauliflower rice, thawed

¼ cup raisins (optional)

1 to 2 tablespoons raw honey (optional)

2 cups plain whole-milk cultured Greek yogurt

1 teaspoon ground cinnamon

2 teaspoons sea salt

MAKES 3 MINI-CAKES OR
1 SMALL LOAF CAKE
Prep time: 10 minutes
Cook time: 25 to 30 minutes

COOKIE DOUGH CAKE

4 large eggs

1 teaspoon baking soda

¾ cup creamy cashew butter

1 teaspoon vanilla extract

1 teaspoon maca powder

Unsweetened chocolate chips,
as desired

Cookie dough is obviously amazing. Cake is surely a go-to. But when you put them together into one, can you make it healthy? Yes, it's a double win! I made this one day on a whim, then tested (and ate) plenty of slices, all without any digestive upsets or the feeling one typically gets after eating sugar-laden cake. This version is light, airy, and free of grains, gluten, dairy, yeast, and sugar (though it oddly still tastes slightly sweet!). A must-make for any occasion!

1   Preheat the oven to 350°F. Grease 3 mini spring-form pans or an 8½ x 4½-inch loaf pan.

2   With an electric or stand mixer, whisk the eggs and baking soda until foamy and doubled in volume. Add the cashew butter, vanilla, and maca powder and continue mixing for a few more minutes.

3   With a spoon, stir in the desired amount of chocolate chips. Pour the batter into the pan(s) and bake for 25 to 30 minutes, or until a toothpick inserted in the center comes out clean.

4   Let cool briefly in the pan, then invert onto a rack to cool completely before serving.

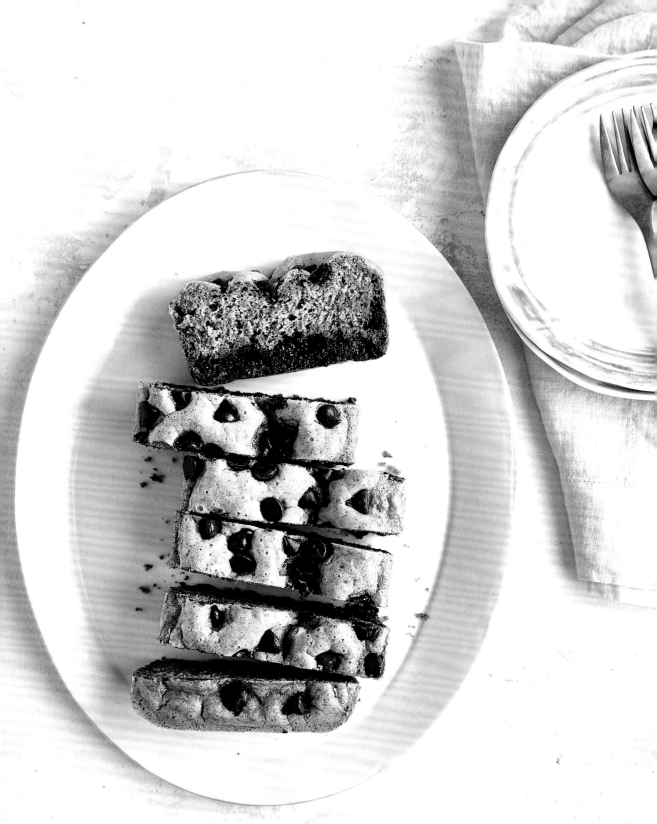

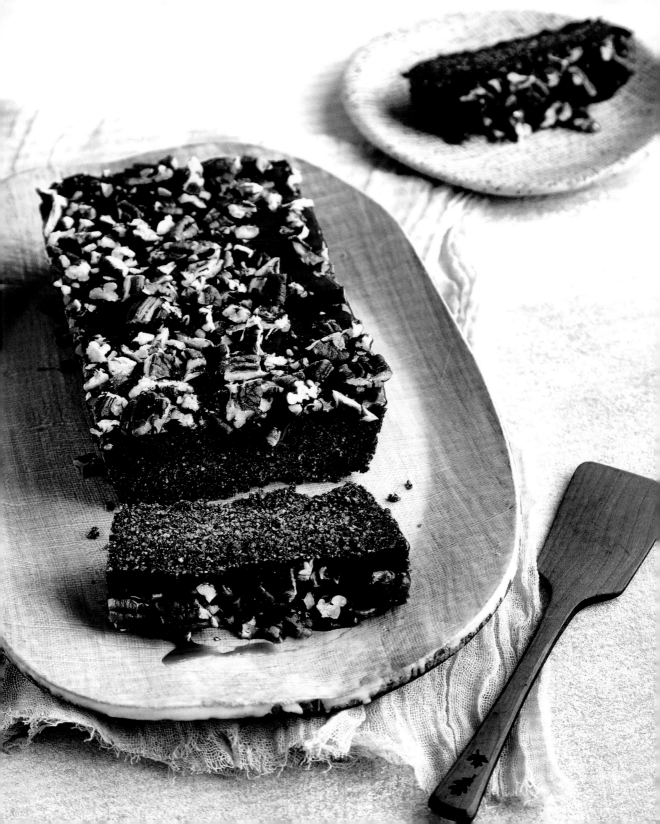

MAKES 1 SMALL LOAF
Prep time: 10 minutes
Cook time: 25 to 30 minutes

PECAN PIE SWEET BREAD

No need to worry about the heaviness of the typical pecan pie in this loaf! The sweetness added is just enough to turn this bread into dessert. And what I love most about it is that the sweetness included is from raw natural honey, which you can adjust to your liking. That's what I love about these loaf recipes. You can always add "extras" after baking—but you can never take away the sweetness once it's added. Customization is key.

1 Preheat the oven to 350°F. Grease an 8½ by 4½-inch loaf pan or line with parchment paper.

2 With an electric or stand mixer, beat the eggs, baking soda, and vinegar for 3 to 4 minutes, until foamy and doubled in volume.

3 Add the pecan flour and coconut flour and continue mixing until the batter is smooth.

4 Pour the batter in the pan and top with some pecan pieces (if desired). Bake for 25 to 30 minutes, or until a toothpick inserted in the center comes out clean.

5 Allow to cool briefly in the pan, then invert onto a rack to cool completely. When cool, drizzle with coconut butter and honey (if using). Better yet, chill the cake in the freezer for 1 hour before drizzling. Store the cake in the refrigerator for up to 5 days or in the freezer up to 2 months.

4 large eggs

1 teaspoon baking soda

1 tablespoon apple cider vinegar

2 cups pecan flour (or 1 cup creamy pecan butter)

¼ cup coconut flour

OPTIONAL TOPPINGS

Pecan pieces

Unsweetened roasted coconut butter (creamed coconut)

Raw honey

MAKES 6 BROWNIES
Prep time: 5 minutes
Cook time: 30 minutes

PRO-BIOTIC VEGAN BROWNIES

1 cup unsweetened applesauce

½ cup (37 grams) chocolate protein powder of choice (such as my Probiotic Cacao Nuzest Protein Powder)

½ cup unsweetened cacao powder

You can't turn down a good brownie. And when they require only three ingredients to make, you really have no excuse *not* to make them! Get your kids involved or call over a friend, rent a movie, and have a baking movie night. These are even delicious the next day cold for breakfast or crumbled on top of a smoothie. So, you're best baking a double batch (trust me, you'll wish you had!).

1   Preheat the oven to 350°F. Line an 8-inch square pan with parchment paper and set aside.

2   In a large bowl, mix all the ingredients until a thick dough forms with the consistency of Play-Doh.

3   Spread the dough in the baking pan, smooth the top, and bake for about 30 minutes, or until a toothpick inserted in the center comes out clean.

4   Allow the brownies to cool completely before cutting into squares. If desired, frost with Best Chocolate Frosting (239).

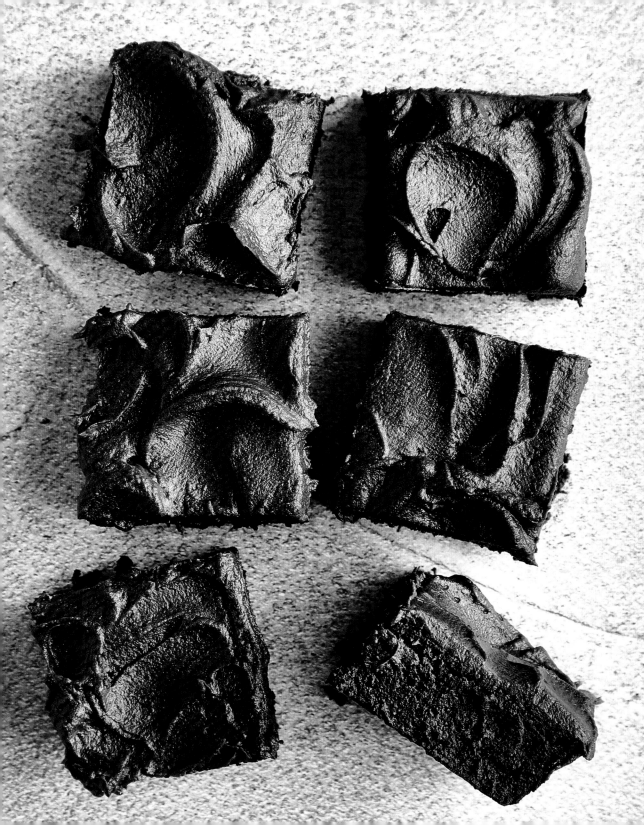

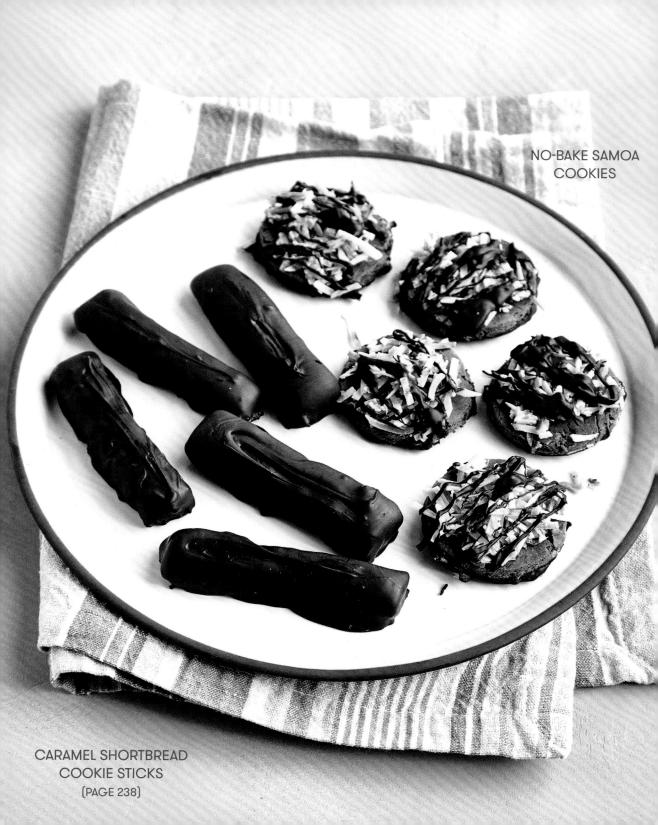

NO-BAKE SAMOA
COOKIES

CARAMEL SHORTBREAD
COOKIE STICKS
(PAGE 238)

NO-BAKE SAMOA COOKIES

I remember eating Girl Scout cookies in my teens, and Samoas were by far my absolute favorite. But of course, all that processed sugar and those chemicals caught up with me in more ways than one, and I haven't had the "real" thing since. But I don't miss them one bit after creating these healthy treats. Honestly, these are an exact replica, but made with only real, wholesome ingredients and loaded with protein! Win–win!

1 Crush the coconut into smaller pieces or crumbs, then mix with the pea protein in a bowl. Add the remaining cookie ingredients and mix until a stiff dough forms.

2 Roll out the dough between two sheets of parchment paper to a thickness of about ¼ inch. Cut into 2-inch diameter circles with a cookie cutter. Place on a baking sheet lined with parchment paper. Place in the freezer to chill while preparing the coconut coating.

3 Mix all coating ingredients; top each cookie with some coating and place back in the freezer to chill.

4 Dip the bottoms of each cookie in the melted chocolate and drizzle the top if desired. Return to the refrigerator to chill. (They also freeze well!)

COOKIE BASE

¼ cup toasted unsweetened shredded coconut

½ cup (37 grams) pea protein powder of choice (such as my Probiotic Vanilla Nuzest Protein Powder)

¼ cup "drippy" almond butter

2 tablespoons unsulfured blackstrap molasses, date syrup, or raw honey

2 tablespoons filtered water

COCONUT COATING

½ cup toasted unsweetened shredded coconut

1 scoop (10 grams) unflavored grass-fed gelatin of choice (such as Vital Proteins)

2 to 3 tablespoons unsulfured blackstrap molasses, date syrup, or raw honey

Unsweetened chocolate, melted, for dipping and drizzle

CARAMEL SHORTBREAD COOKIE STICKS

1 cup pitted Medjool dates, soaked in warm water for 20 minutes and drained

1 tablespoon organic SunButter (or creamy nut or seed butter of choice)

1 tablespoon coconut butter (creamed coconut), melted

1 teaspoon sea salt

1 recipe Carb-Free Crumb Cookies (page 226), made without the chocolate chips, shaped into a single layer instead of circles, and baked, then placed in freezer to chill

Unsweetened chocolate, for coating

The familiar Twix candy bars bring me back to summers spent listening to the free summer concerts in the park. We all have those memories that certain foods evoke, and Twix certainly brings many back to my mind. Perhaps that's why they hold a special place in my heart? Or perhaps it's just because they are so dang delicious! Ha! Whatever the case may be for you, I hope this healthy remake recalls a special memory and also creates some new ones!

1   Place the dates in warm water to cover and soak to plump up briefly.

2   Drain the water from the dates and blend them with the SunButter, melted coconut butter, and sea salt until smooth (the smaller the blender the better—a bullet blender works well).

3   Remove the cookie layer from the freezer and spread the caramel evenly over it. Place the cookie layer back in the freezer to chill the caramel.

4   Melt the coating chocolate. Remove the cookie layer from the freezer and slice into desired shapes, then coat each piece with the melted chocolate. Store the cookies in the refrigerator for up to 3 days or in the freezer for up to 1 month.

MAKES 1½ CUPS
Prep time: 10 minutes
Chill time: 5 hours

THE BEST CHOCOLATE FROSTING

Frosting you can eat by the spoon? I'm in! You can also use this frosting to top cupcakes, cakes, and pancakes, or as a fruit dip, or smeared on a slice of your Best Basic Sandwich Bread (page 103). The possibilities are endless!

½ cup unsweetened chocolate, melted

1½ cups sweet potato puree (see Note)

½ teaspoon ground cinnamon

¼ teaspoon vanilla extract

1   Place the chocolate, sweet potato puree, cinnamon, and vanilla in a blender and blend until smooth.

2   Refrigerate for at least 5 hours or overnight to allow the frosting to thicken to a firm "icing-like" consistency. Store in the refrigerator for up to 5 days.

NOTE: Peel the potatoes and then steam until tender and puree. Or, substitute canned sweet potato.

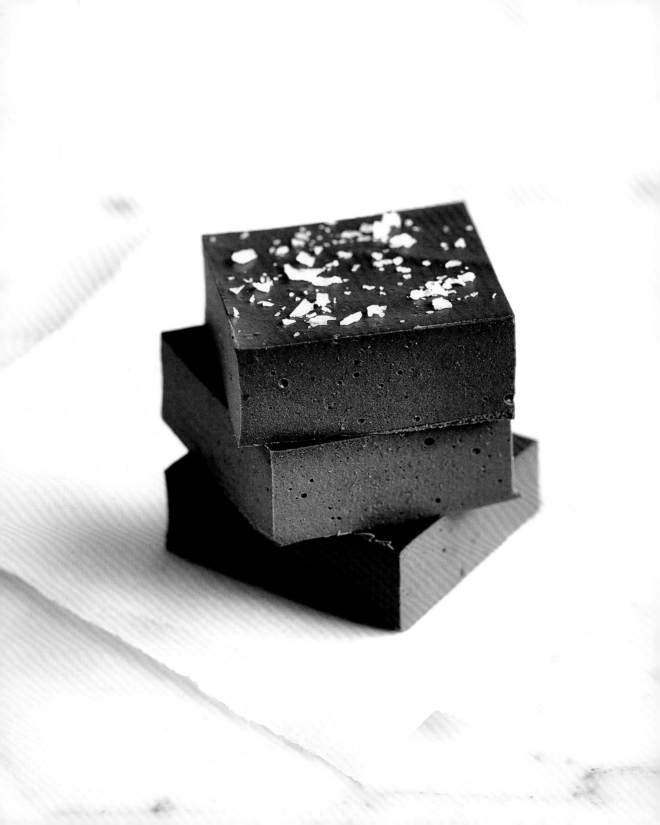

MAKES 8 OUNCES OF FUDGE
Prep time: 5 minutes
Cook time: 1 hour
Chill time: 1 to 2 hours

SEA SALT BUTTER- NUT FUDGE

Ever order fudge at a county fair? You know, those booths where you can order by the pound? As a kid, I always begged my mom every time we walked the fairgrounds, and I was lucky to get a small square. Today, if I eat a square of fudge I get a huge headache from all the refined sugar. (It's crazy how our bodies change and adjust after detoxing!) But that doesn't mean I don't crave fudge. These healthy squares honestly hit the spot, without bad effects! They are naturally sweet from the butternut squash, contain loads of gut-healing gelatin and healthy fats, and leave your sweet tooth feeling satisfied.

1   Preheat the oven to 350°F. Line an 8½ x 4½-inch loaf pan with parchment paper.

2   Puree the coconut oil, coconut butter, cocoa powder, dates, salt, and gelatin in a blender until smooth. Add the squash puree and blend with the remaining ingredients (do not add any liquid) until smooth.

3   Pour the mixture into the prepared pan and refrigerate about 2 to 3 hours, or until firm. Cut into bite-size pieces and enjoy.

¼ cup coconut oil

2 tablespoons coconut butter (creamed coconut)

½ cup unsweetened cocoa powder

2 Medjool dates, pitted

1 teaspoon sea salt

2½ scoops (25 grams) unflavored grass-fed gelatin of choice (such as Vital Proteins)

1 medium butternut squash, baked and flesh scooped out (about 1 cup pureed)

LOW-CARB BUTTERNUT BROWNIES

For those looking for a lower-carb, lower-sugar brownie that's vegan and Paleo, look no further! Made with cacao protein powder and winter squash, these moist squares of bliss are perfect for any occasion, any time of the year (thankfully, butternut squash is available all year long).

1 cup butternut squash puree (or sweet potato or pumpkin puree)

½ cup (37 grams) chocolate protein powder of choice (such as my Probiotic Cacao Nuzest Protein Powder)

½ cup unsweetened cocoa powder

¼ cup fine flax meal (grind flax meal in a small bullet blender until super fine)

Unsweetened chocolate chips to top, as desired (optional)

1   Preheat the oven to 350°F. Line an 8-inch baking pan with parchment paper or grease a cupcake tin.

2   Mix all the ingredients except the chocolate chips in a large bowl until well blended. Spread the dough in the baking pan or spoon into the cupcake molds. Press down firmly. (Note: This batter does not rise, so you can fill the pan to the desired height.)

3   Bake for about 30 minutes, or until a toothpick inserted in the center comes out clean. Immediately top the brownies with some chocolate chips (if using), then allow to cool completely before cutting into squares. Store in the refrigerator for up to 3 days or freeze for up to 3 weeks.

NO-BAKE PROBIOTIC CHOCOLATE CHEESECAKE

Did you ever hide food in your fridge so no one else in the house ate it? Guilty! This cake is definitely one of those "place in the back of the refrigerator so no one sees it" types of cakes. But sharing is caring, right? I mean, you can always make two!

½ cup unsweetened chocolate, melted

1½ cups cultured cottage cheese

½ cup raisins, soaked in warm water for 10 minutes and drained

2 scoops (20 grams) unflavored grass-fed gelatin of choice (such as Vital Proteins)

Shavings of unsweetened chocolate, for garnish

1   Line a 4-inch mini springform pan or mold with parchment paper or use a silicone mold.

2   Place the melted chocolate, cottage cheese, and raisins in a blender and blend until creamy.

3   Add the gelatin and blend for an additional 30 seconds.

4   Pour the mixture into the prepared pan. Smooth the top, and top with the chocolate shavings. Chill in the refrigerator for 45 minutes, or until cake is set. When ready to serve, slice the cake and enjoy. Store in the refrigerator for up to 4 days.

Three-Ingredient
(VEGAN) FUDGE

3 medium ripe, spotty bananas

½ cup unsweetened cocoa powder

½ cup coconut butter (creamed coconut), melted

Easy recipes are made more often, agreed? Especially when they actually taste good! With only three simple, every-day ingredients, this is one of those "make weekly" kind of desserts.

Place the bananas, cocoa powder, and coconut butter in a blender and blend until everything is silky smooth. Transfer to a small dish lined with wax paper and freeze for 30 to 60 minutes or until firm, or refrigerate overnight. Slice and enjoy! Store in the refrigerator for up to 4 days or freeze for up to 1 month.

APPENDIX: SELECTED RESEARCH

IT'S NOT IN YOUR HEAD— IT'S YOUR GUT

Pimentel, M., Morales, W., Rezale, A., Marsh, E., Lembo, A., Mirocha, J., et al. (2015). "Development and Validation of a Biomarker for Diarrhea-Predominant Irritable Bowel Syndrome in Human Subjects." *PLoS ONE* 10(5): e0126438.

Pimentel, M. (July 2016). "A Predictive Model to Estimate Cost Savings of a Novel Diagnostic Blood Panel for Diagnosis of Diarrhea-Predominant Irritable Bowel Syndrome." *Clinical Therapeutics* 38(7): 1638–1652.

Klem, F., et al. (April 2017). "Prevalence, Risk Factors, and Outcomes of Irritable Bowel Syndrome After Infectious Enteritis: A Systematic Review and Meta-Analysis." *Gastroenterology* 152(5): 1042–1054.

National Institute of Diabetes and Digestive Diseases. (November 2017). "Symptoms & Causes of Irritable Bowel Syndrome." www.niddk.nih.gov/health-information/digestive-diseases /irritable-bowel-syndrome/symptoms-causes.

National Center for Complementary and Integrative Health. (September 24, 2017). "4 Fast Facts about the Gut-Brain Connection." nccih.nih.gov/news/events/IMlectures/gut -brain.

National Institutes of Health. (October 2, 2018). "Gut Communicates Directly with Brain." www.nih.gov/news-events /nih-research-matters/gut-communicates-directly-brain.

Allergan and Gastrointestinal Society. (2018). "IBS Global Impact Report." badgut.org/wp-content/uploads/IBS -Global-Impact-Report.pdf.

Gastrointestinal Society. (2016). "Survey Results: Irritable Bowel Syndrome." badgut.org/wp-content/uploads/IBS -Survey-Results-2016.pdf.

International Foundation for Gastrointestinal Disorders. (June 1, 2017). "Gut Bacteria and IBS." www.aboutibs.org /gut-bacteria-and-ibs.html.

National Center for Health Statistics. (January 19, 2017). "Therapeutic Drug Use." www.cdc.gov/nchs/fastats /drug-use-therapeutic.htm.

YOUR GUT, FROM THE INSIDE OUT: DEBUNKING DIGESTIVE HEALTH MYTHS

Patel, A., et al. (May 30, 2016). "Effects of Disturbed Sleep on Gastrointestinal and Somatic Pain Symptoms in IBS." *Alimentary & Pharmacology Therapeutics.* 44(3): 246–258.

Goldsmith, G., and Levin, J. (October 1993). "Effect of Sleep Quality on Symptoms of Irritable Bowel Syndrome." *Digest of Digestive Sciences* 38(10): 1809–1814.

Xiong, W., et al. (June 4, 2012). "Cannabinoids Suppress Inflammatory and Neuropathic Pain by Targeting α3 Glycine Receptors." *Journal of Experimental Medicine* 209(6): 1121–1134.

Schier, A. R., et al. (June 2012). "Cannabidiol, a Cannabis Sativa Constituent, as an Anxiolytic Drug." *Brazilian Journal of Psychiatry* 34 (Suppl. 1): S104–110.

DiPatrizio, N. (2016). "Endocannabinoids in the Gut." *Cannabis and Cannabinoid Research* 1(1): 67–77.

Qorri, B., et al. (October 12, 2017). "Preventing Negative Shifts in Gut Microbiota with Cannabis Therapy: Implications for Colorectal Cancer." *Advanced Research in Gastroenterology and Hepatology* 10.19080/ARGH.2017.07.555712.

Di Carlo, G., and Izzo, A. (March 2, 2005). "Cannabinoids for Gastrointestinal Diseases: Potential Therapeutic Applications." *Expert Opinion on Investigational Drugs.* doi .org/10.1517/13543784.12.1.39.

Hornby, P., and Prouty, S. (April 4, 2004). "Involvement of Cannabinoid Receptors in Gut Motility and Visceral Perception." *British Journal of Pharmacology* 141(8): 1335–1345.

Berkey, C., et al. (June 2005). "Milk, Dairy Fat, Dietary Calcium, and Weight Gain: A Longitudinal Study of Adolescents." *Archives of Pediatric and Adolescent Medicine* 159(6): 543–550.

National Institute of Diabetes and Digestive and Kidney Diseases. (December 2017). "Your Digestive System & How It Works." www.niddk.nih.gov/health-information /digestive-diseases/digestive-system-how-it-works.

Nugent, A. P. (February 16, 2005). "Health Properties of Resistant Starch." *Nutrition Bulletin*. https://doi.org/10.1111 /j.1467-3010.2005.00481.x.

Englyst, H. N., et al. (May 1996). "Measurement of Resistant Starch in Vitro and in Vivo." *British Journal of Nutrition* 75(5): 749-755.

21 DAYS TO A HEALTHY GUT: THE GUT RESET

Roxas, M. (December 2008). "The Role of Enzyme Supplementation in Digestive Disorders." *Alternative Medicine Review* 13(4): 307-314.

Brien, S., et al. (December 2004). "Bromelain as a Treatment for Osteoarthritis: A Review of Clinical Studies." *Evidence-Based Complementary and Alternative Medicine* 1(3): 247-251

Muhammed, Z., and Ahmad, T. (January 2017). "Therapeutic Uses of Pineapple-Extracted Bromelain in Surgical Care—A Review." *Journal of the Pakistani Medical Association* 67(1): 121-125.

Muss, C., et al. (2013). "Papaya Preparation (Caricol®) in Digestive Disorders." *Neuro Endocrinology Letters* 34(1): 38-46.

Kaur, L., and Boland, M. (2013). "Influence of Kiwifruit on Protein Digestion." *Advanced Food and Nutrition Research* 68: 149-167. doi: 10.1016/B978-0-12-394294-4.00008-0.

AFTER THE GUT RESET: ENJOYING YOUR HEALTHY GUT—FOR LIFE

Bonnema, A., et al. (June 2010). "Gastrointestinal Tolerance of Chicory Inulin Products." *Journal of the American Dietetic Association* 110(6): 865-868. doi: 10.1016/j .jada.2010.03.025.

Ripoll, C., et al. (July-August 2010). "Gastrointestinal Tolerance to an Inulin-Rich Soluble Roasted Chicory Extract After Consumption in Healthy Subjects." *Nutrition* 26(7-8): 799-803. doi: 10.1016/j.nut.2009.07.013.

Bacchetta, J., et al. (October 2008). "Renal Hypersensitivity to Inulin and IgA Nephropathy." *Pediatric Nephrology* 23(10): 1883-1885. doi: 10.1007/s00467-008-0819-9.

ACKNOWLEDGMENTS

This book would not have been possible without the unfailing love and continued support from my parents, Tim and Becky Ugarte. They were there with me while I was deathly ill, while I healed, and encouraged me to keep pushing forward until I was healthy again and inspired me to share my knowledge and experience with the masses through a book. They were my backbone, and words or material things will never express how grateful I am for their support.

My writer, Kelly James, put onto paper what I could only express through verbiage. She could read my thoughts and knew exactly what I was thinking and wanted to say before saying it. I could not have asked for a better, more perfect person to help me organize this book so perfectly and lead me through each step along the way as a first-time author. Her talent is beyond extraordinary and I would've been lost without her!

And what would a book be without beautiful photos? That's where my photographer, Hélène Dujardin, deserves major credit! She brought my recipes to life and captured every detail while I stood by her side. She not only holds incredible talent, but her southern hospitality while I visited her studio for the photoshoot will stick with me forever.

The team at Crown Publishing, specifically Diana Baroni and Michele Eniclerico, and my managers Steve Troha and Dado Derviskadic from Folio Literacy were the perfect group to lead on this book and conduct all the loose ends. I couldn't have asked for a better team to bring this dream to life!

Mohammad Nikkhah was THE holistic doctor that literally saved my life. He never gave up on me while I was ill and was the one who opened my eyes to the true meaning of health. If it wasn't for him, I don't think I would have made it. He has a heart of gold, keeps me humble, and I still love learning from him to this day!

God is *really* the One who deserves all the praise. He is truly the one who saved me and sent all the above people into my life to get me where I am today. Lastly mentioned, but certainly not the least. . . . God truly deserves all the praise and His name will forever be glorified.

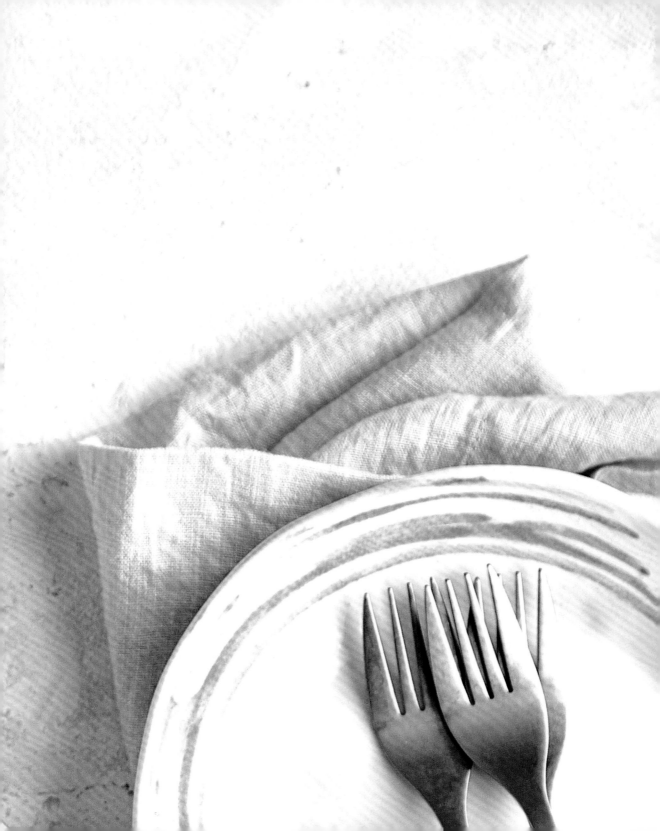

INDEX

Note: Page numbers in *italics* indicate recipes.

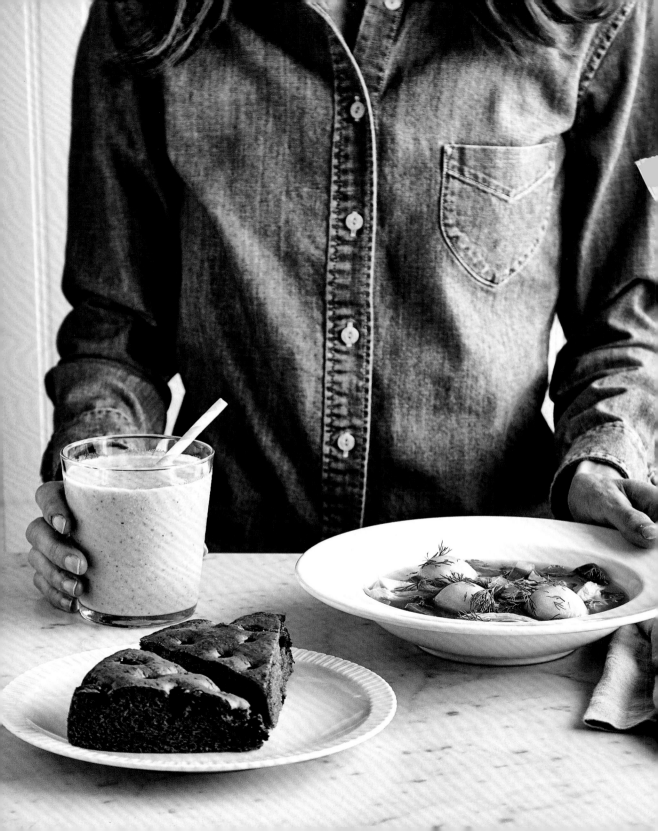